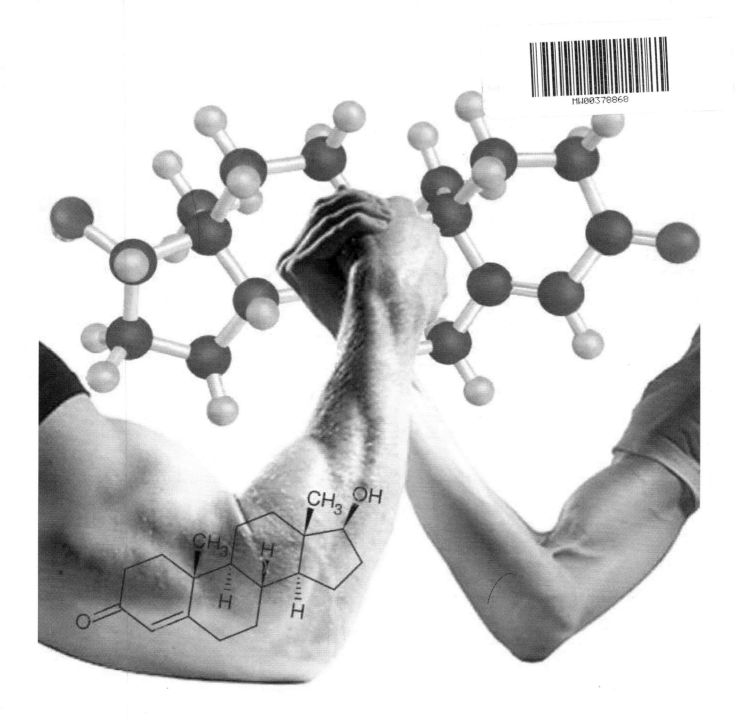

UPGRADE Your Testosterone
UPGRADE Your Health

By Logan Christopher
www.LegendaryStrength.com

DISCLAIMER

The exercises and training information contained within this book may be too strenuous or dangerous for some people, and the reader should consult with a physician before engaging in them. The health advice contained within this book is for educational purposes only and is not intended for medical purposes. Please see your doctor before making any changes to your diet or lifestyle.

The author and publisher of this book are not responsible in any manner whatsoever for the use, misuse or dis-use of the information presented here.

All images, unless otherwise noted, are from my private collection. They are reproduced here under the professional practice of fair use for the purposes of historical discussion and scholarly interpretation. All characters and images remain the property of their respective copyright holders.

Published by:
Legendary Strength LLC.
Santa Cruz, California

www.LegendaryStrength.com

Table of Contents

Introduction to the Upgrade Your Health Series

Upgrade Your Health is all about taking where you're currently at with one aspect of your health and bringing it up to a higher level. It's not a matter of doing it wrong, or doing it right. While some things are clearly bad or clearly good, this isn't a game of black and white. Instead there are many shades of grey. There is lots of room for better or worse. Sometimes there will be a best and worst, but when you look at that, the answer can be malleable and changing over time, especially when it comes to you as an individual.

Ideally, you'd want to be at the top end of the spectrum, but for a variety of reasons you may not be able to get there immediately. If you can, great, make that leap. But even if you can just climb one rung up the ladder, that step will improve your health. Then after some time you can make the next step, and so on, until you reach the top.

In some cases there may not always be a clear answer on what is the best. And since everyone is individual you have to experiment and find what works best for you and your lifestyle.

Either way, by taking the incremental approach, or the big leap to betterment, you can work towards the goal of "Radiant Health". I first heard of this Daoist idea from one of my teachers, Ron Teeguarden. The idea behind this is that you reach a place of "health beyond danger". That means a place where sickness and disease cannot effect you. It's a good place to be at! So how do you get there? By upgrading all the different areas of health.

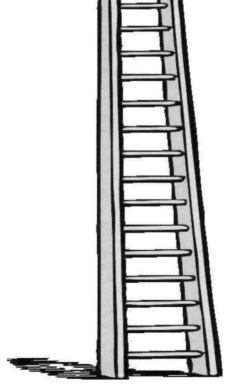

Unfortunately it's not as simple as take this pill, or eat this, not that. There's much more to health than that. And I would argue that the majority of people are spending too much time on the wrong things. For instance, what you eat, while important, isn't the whole picture. The truth is if you upgrade every other area of health then what you eat won't be that important. And doing so can be both fun and easy to do. It can become a challenging exploration that gives you bountiful rewards.

Furthermore, by upgrading your health you can also upgrade your performance. By having all of your bodily systems working for you, rather than against you, you'll find that gaining strength, skill and the body you desire becomes much easier to do. By doing all the things that best support your health you'll find your body will automatically move towards looking its best. This is because form follows function. Optimize the function of your systems and "the system" will look and work great.

Your energy will improve. So will your cognition and your ability to be productive and hit any goal you desire. Great health is one thing many successful people have in common.

Most of what we focus on in this series could be called the basics. However as you'll come to see, there are lots of details that can go into these basics. We'll dive deep into each topic giving you every detail I can give from all of my research and personal experimentation to help you upgrade where you're at.

In my earlier books *101 Simple Steps to Radiant Health* and *101 Advanced Steps to Radiant Health*, I delivered a bunch of tips to upgrade your health. While there may be a collection of tips on a specific topic, it wasn't structured in a way like this series is designed to be. Here you can dive into one topic deeply to bring it to the next level.

Yet looking with this much detail can often be overwhelming. But by diving into this detailed view then zooming back out to the bigger picture we can learn many things that we can then implement into our lives. As always this guide ends with a condensed action plan of what to do to really upgrade this area of your health. So without further ado…

The Importance of Testosterone

Testosterone is one of the most important hormones in the human body. It is used by both men and women, though men have roughly 7-8 times the testosterone as an adult, over children. And 20 times the daily production, about 4 to 7 milligrams a day, than women do. Estrogen is considered the female hormone equivalent, which males have as well, just in smaller amounts. At least typically. With endocrine disruption in both men and women, in older age many men can have higher estrogen levels than their wives.

Testosterone is the hormone, along with the other androgens, that makes men men. The word testosterone was coined by Dutch professor Ernst Laqueur in 1923 and we've been talking about it ever since. When a fetus is developing in the second trimester, a surge of testosterone is what causes the dividing cells to become male instead of female. More surges occur shortly after being born, and of course, the most well-known, during puberty.

A deficiency of testosterone has been linked to the following issues:

- Depression
- Inability to Focus, Concentrate and Remember
- Anxiety
- Increased Fat especially in the Abdomen
- Decreased Libido
- Erectile Dysfunction
- Reduced Muscle Mass and Strength
- Balding
- Osteoporosis
- Dry Skin
- Increased Risk of Cardiovascular Disease, Stroke and Heart Attacks
- Accelerated Aging
- Aches and Pains
- Excessive Sweating
- Irritability or Anger
- Fatigue

Contrast this to the benefits of high testosterone. As an anabolic substance, testosterone causes increased protein synthesis allowing for faster and better recovery, which leads to increased muscle mass as well and increased bone density. Its role in sex is obvious and it may be even more important for attitude as it acts as a neurohormone. High testosterone gives you the feeling that you can *"Take on the World"*.

For this reason optimizing testosterone has become an important part of not just performance but for health in all areas.

Testosterone-replacement therapy (TRT) is an FDA approved method administered by doctors to help older men restore youthful levels of testosterone. While it has brought benefits to many, it's also been linked to increased strokes, heart attacks and death. The risk and benefits need to be weighed. In any case, I believe it is best to first work with more natural means to boost your endogenous testosterone, meaning the testosterone your body produces, rather than from external sources. Directly injected testosterone leads to dependence on it, shutting down your own body's production. It also acts a Band-Aid, rather than fixing the issues that have caused your body to slow production of its own testosterone.

Besides testosterone is just one of a symphony of hormones that is important. If you only add in one, that doesn't necessarily fix any of the other issues. But working on it naturally you tend to get a more holistic increase, thus the natural approach is what this book is about.

Andropause is the male equivalent to the female menopause. Female menopause occurs in a limited age range of 45-55. Andropause on the other hand can begin in the 30's though it generally is at its peak around 50 as well.

Another term you may see is "Estrogen Dominance Syndrome" as the problems with low testosterone are not just about the androgens, but an excess of estrogen.

With even more of an estrogenic environment, and the younger generations, starting out with it from before birth, I wouldn't be surprised if men in their 20's start seeing andropause symptoms either. As a baby is bathed in these chemicals before they're even born, this could have more devastating impact in the future. Studies have shown that overall testosterone levels are dropping in men, not just with age, as you can see in this chart.

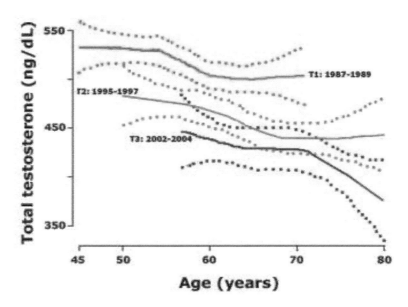

The good news is that this is largely within your control if you're willing to put in the work. *Upgrade Your Testosterone* will take a deep look at the complexity of our hormonal system and the several different steps you'll have to take to optimize it.

Side Note for Women

This book is meant for men primarily. It's simply that I am a man and work mostly with men. Plus female hormones are significantly more complex then men's. If you want something directed towards females I recommend reading *The Hormone Cure* from Dr. Sara Gottfried as a decent starting place.

That being said, as we focus on natural approaches, much of the information here will work wonders for women as well to help regulate their hormones too. As with everything, take what is useful and discard the rest.

Lifelong Testosterone Insufficiency

Testosterone is an important subject to me for a few reasons. As I've focused my life and career on strength and health, with hormone function being intimately tied into those, I have sought out what can be done to have better testosterone levels.

Part of this may stem from the fact that it hasn't come easy to me. Apparently I've suffered from "lifelong testosterone insufficiency". This means that since being conceived, probably before I left the womb, I've had less testosterone than the average person.

I didn't have blood work as a child so I can't give you numbers, but based on a few observations I believe this to be the case. I was a frail and weakly child. I often got sick. When I entered high school I weighed 98 pounds, and didn't seem to hit puberty quite as well as other people.

As other guys sprouted hair all over, I really didn't. I can remember being embarrassed in the locker rooms to have so little armpit hair. Still to this day I have zero hair on my chest. And my facial hair is slow growing and spotty. I was able to grow my first beard at 30 and it's still far from great.

As Dr. Malcolm Carruthers says in his book, *Testosterone Revolution*, "Although the amount of hair on the chest is also hereditary, it is affected by lifelong testosterone levels. Sometimes, if it is very much reduced and the man only has to shave once or twice a week, it can indicate a life-long insufficiency of this hormone."

Further, I wasn't as sexual as others my age. A lot of this was psychological and social, but those issues likely stemmed from the lack of testosterone as well.

I'm the third of three children. My two brothers did not have the same issues as I did. As pointed out in *Deep Nutrition*, Dr. Shanahan says that if a mother (with the father contributing as well) is not getting the right nutrition, and spacing her babies out, it can lead to some health issues.

If you look at the Chinese medicine model of the three treasures, I would be considered as having less *jing* than others. There is most definitely a big hormonal component to the *jing* energy.

This is all to say that genetically, my baseline, was not to be a high testosterone male. Thus, to get to this position, I've had to do a lot more work than most probably would. And I probably have to be more exact in what I do on a regular basis in order to stay there.

The good news is that there is a lot that can be done, even if you're in a case like mine, or even worse off.

How Testosterone, and about 20 Other Hormones, are Created and Converted

Before we look at what you can do, it's important to have a general understanding of testosterone production and the many other hormones at play. Warning: this is science. Although I try to avoid too many big words, besides the names of the components we're talking about, it may still be overwhelming on first view. That's okay. Just a general understanding will help, and even if you skip this part, you can still take action to increase your testosterone later on.

We begin with the names of hormones and other important components, as well as their abbreviations. These will be mentioned once again during the text for ease of use.

- Gonadotropin-releasing Hormone (GnRH)
- Follicle-Stimulating Hormone (FSH)
- Luteinizing Hormone (LH)
- Androgen-binding protein (ABP)
- Cholesterol
- Pregnenolone (P5)
- Progesterone (P4)
- Dehydroepiandrosterone (DHEA)
- Androstenedione
- Androstenediol
- Testosterone (T)
- Dihydrotestosterone (DHT)
- Androstenol
- Androstenone
- Estrone (E1)
- Estradiol (E2)
- Estriol (E3)
- Cortisol
- Prolactin (PRL)
- Sex Hormone Binding Globulin (SHBG)
- Albumin
- Free Testosterone (Free-T)

It all starts with the hypothalamus, the master hormone signaler in the brain. Actually there are feedback loops so you can't really say it "starts" anywhere. The body senses when testosterone (T) is low, which triggers the release of gonadotropin-releasing hormone (GnRH). This occurs in several pulses throughout the day. It operates on a negative feedback loop, becoming inhibited once T is aromatized into estradiol (E2) which decreases responsiveness to GnRH.

GnRH then triggers the pituitary gland, another gland in the brain, to produce two hormones, luteinizing hormone (LH) and follicle-stimulating hormone (FSH), which then travel down to the testicles. FSH increases the production of androgen-binding protein (ABP) in the testes. ABP, as the name implies, binds to T, DHT and E2. Its primary job is in spermatogenesis, which is the production of sperm. FSH's main role is in the ability to procreate.

LH starts the production of testosterone, through a long chain of conversions. Thus, LH is responsible for pregnenolone, androstenedione, DHEA and others, in what are known as the Leydig cells.

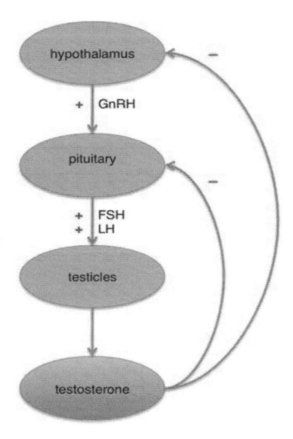

All steroid hormones originally come from cholesterol. This is reason enough for getting sufficient cholesterol from your diet, which comes mostly from animal fats. However the human body can also produce its own cholesterol in the liver. The Leydig cells can synthesize cholesterol from acetyl coenzyme A or use up low density lipoprotein (LDL, the "bad" cholesterol) that's floating around. The Leydig cells make the conversions from cholesterol to testosterone using five different enzymes over a series of steps.

Cholesterol is converted into pregnenolone (P5) which can then be converted in DHEA, through an intermediary step. DHEA is the most common circulating steroid hormone in the human body. It's created in the gonads, adrenal glands and brain, and can further be transformed into other androgens. DHEA has very weak androgenic properties itself. The sulfated form, DHEA-S, is what is normally measured in the body.

Pregnenolone is also converted into progesterone (P4). This occurs in the testicles. Pregnenolone and DHEA have many benefits beyond the scope of this book. While progesterone is important for men, it is even more so for women, where it is the primary hormone that modulates estrogen.

DHEA can be converted into androstenedione, which can then be converted into testosterone or estrone (E1). DHEA also converts into androstenediol, which converts into testosterone. Both of these two hormones, coming from DHEA, have weak androgenic properties themselves.

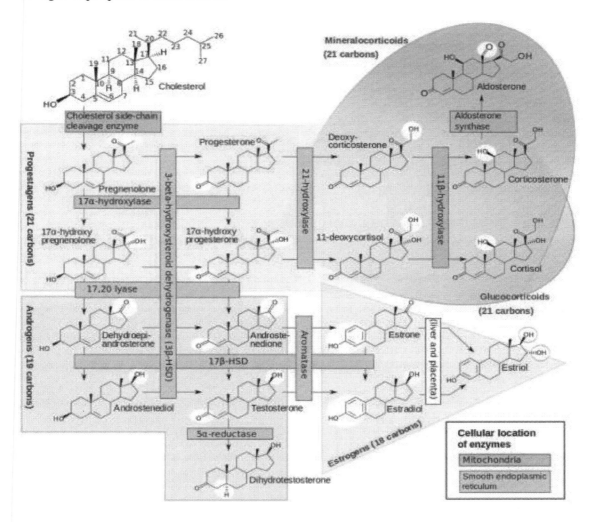

Around 95% of testosterone is produced by testicles in men. Women produce it in the ovaries. Much smaller amounts of testosterone, about 5%, are also produced in the adrenal glands. It's important to note that testosterone and androstenedione convert back and forth between each other relying on a zinc-dependent enzyme, 17-beta-hydroxysteroid dehydrogenase.

Testosterone can be converted into dihydrotestosterone (DHT) via enzyme 5a-reductase, or aromatized into estradiol (E2). In men, approximately 5% of T is converted into DHT, which is an even more potent androgen, with somewhere around 5 to 50 times the biological activity, depending on who you ask. Furthermore, DHT cannot be aromatized into estrogen.

Excessive DHT is linked to male pattern baldness and was previously thought to contribute to benign prostatic hyperplasia (BPH), but since that time this has become known to be more a function of excess estrogen.

Unfortunately, not a whole lot is known about all these conversions. For instance, zinc, as will be described in detail later, is well known to be critical for testosterone production. It is needed to convert androstenedione to testosterone. However, it's probably used in several other conversions in this cycle as well. All kinds of other vitamins, minerals and other cofactors are undoubtedly needed too.

Testosterone is also broken down into androstenone and androstenol which are two pheromones. Yes, all these "andro's" start to sound the same, but note that these are different from the previous ones. And these are not shown on the above chart. These are released in the scrotum, armpits and urine. In fact, androstenone gives the characteristic smell of male urine.

But it doesn't end there. Aromatization is the conversion of androgens into estrogens. This occurs via the enzyme aromatase. If you're looking for the benefits of more testosterone this is one of the things that can get in the way. Although primarily a class of female hormones, men have estrogen too, just in lower amounts. Estrogenic activity tends to disrupt androgenic activity, so in general smaller amounts are good. This is one of the primary areas of importance for optimizing testosterone.

Estrone (E1) is synthesized from androstenedione via aromatase.

Estradiol (E2) is synthesized from testosterone via aromatase. This is the primary estrogen that is looked at in male blood tests. This is because if your testosterone is being aromatized than it's not being used for its androgenic effects and can lead to excess estrogen. But estradiol, in the right amount, is necessary. Some of its functions include maintaining the neurotransmitter acetylcholine, supporting healthy sexual function, blood flow, skin health and more.

Estriol (E3) is converted over from both E1 and E2 and not directly from androgens. Its range tends not to increase or decrease that much in men.

For our purposes of optimizing hormones, for most men this will include lowering estrogen. It's important to note that estrogen cannot be converted back into the androgens.

Even when we have testosterone, and it's not being converted into estrogen it can become bound up and unusable. Most of this testosterone becomes bound by sex hormone-binding globulin (SHBG) or albumin, while a small amount, generally 3-5%, circulates freely. Free-T is more important for androgenic qualities than Total T, though for optimal hormone health you want good levels of both. The ratio of total testosterone to SHBG is often called the free androgen index.

SHBG favors hormones in this order, DHT, T, androstenediol, E2, E1. DHEA is weakly bound to SHBG but the other form, DHEA-S, is not bound at all. Note that SHBG has a higher affinity for the androgens than for the estrogens. The role of SHBG is in transporting these hormones around the body. However, once it grabs hold, it tends not to want to let go.

The other main protein that binds to testosterone is albumin. Unlike SHBG though, the link between these two is weak and can be separated easier so this bound testosterone is more bioavailable.

There's also the corticosteroid side of this picture. You'll see that there are several types of cortisol molecules, but we'll keep this simple and just talk about cortisol, which is known as the "stress hormone". While it gets a bad name because we often have too much of it, cortisol has crucial functions within the body. You'll notice that these are created from pregnenolone and progesterone. What happens is, with too much stress, and thus the need for more cortisol, this can "steal" away much of the precursor material, and thus inhibit testosterone function.

Another hormone that plays into this mix is prolactin (PRL). Prolactin was first associated with the production of breast milk, hence the name (pro-lactation), but it has far more uses, the current count being over 300 in the human body regulating metabolism, immune function and more. Prolactin has to do with sexual gratification, countering the effects of dopamine, and is thought to be responsible for the sexual refractory period in men, that is not being able to have sex immediately after having ejaculation. Excessive amounts are thought to be responsible for impotence and lack of libido as it counteracts dopamine, necessary for arousal. In addition, high levels of prolactin decrease sex hormones, possibly by suppressing GnRH.

Another large issue that can come into play, though often not discussed, is with the androgen receptors on cells. These may become less responsive due to a number of factors. Just like there is insulin resistance which occurs before full diabetes, there is androgen resistance. Thus making sure that the receptors and your cells are healthy is another area we'll look at.

As you can see, even though male hormones are much simpler than women's, they're still complex. Women's hormones alternate significantly over a monthly cycle. Men have a cycle too, but it operates daily without big shifts over the course of a month. Testosterone follows a daily rhythm that peaks early each day in the morning. It continues to go down after this time, though there are different pulses of it throughout the day.

If you're looking to optimize your testosterone, you can see that this has to do with a complex interplay of many other hormones. Thus it takes a multi-prong approach. This is why no single solution will work for everyone. That's why we'll try to cover every possible angle.

The Testosterone Metaphor

Now that we've covered the science of how these hormones convert and react with each other, it's important to take a step back and look at the bigger picture. By understanding the symbolic and metaphorical nature of nature you'll have a greater understanding of how it all fits together.

A lot of this came to me in a flash of insight while meditating on testosterone. It tied together the whole picture, giving meaning to all the science I had been diving into. The science is great, and we'll get back to much more of that, but it must be anchored in a bigger vision and even philosophy to really make much sense.

The word hormone comes from the Greek verb *hormao*, meaning "to put into quick motion, to excite or to arouse." Hormones are known as the chemical messengers in the body. As messengers they work to communicate from one area of the body to another.

It's interesting to look at the dual nature of these. Which comes first, the chicken or the egg? It's a paradox with hormones too, because the messengers appear to work in both directions.

The desire and ability to have sex is dependent on testosterone, among other things. And yet, having sex also boosts testosterone. Studies show that even watching sex, live at a sex club or with porn, increases testosterone, though not as much as engaging in it.

Testosterone helps to add muscle and even bone mass by itself. So does strength training. So we see that working out boosts testosterone, but you're also more likely to be active and work out when T is high.

When you look at this you realize you have more control. **If you send the right messages the hormones will respond.**

A recent study looked at body language and testosterone and found that by taking more "dominant" poses testosterone immediately increased while and cortisol went down. And the opposite occurred in "non-dominant" poses raising cortisol and lowering testosterone. Similar hormone effects have been noted in wild animals between the alpha males and beta males.

Just what are those high-power and low-power poses? See for yourself on the next page. And then take a look at how you are right now reading this…

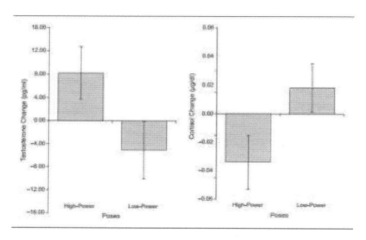

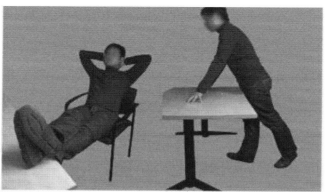

Fig. 1. The two high-power poses used in the study. Participants in the high-power-pose condition were posed in expansive positions with open limbs.

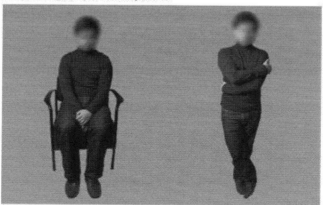

Fig. 2. The two low-power poses used in the study. Participants in the low-power-pose condition were posed in contractive positions with closed limbs.

In neuro-linguistic programming (NLP) it's commonly pointed out that your physiology, that is your posture and movements, determines your state and internal representations, which basically means how you think and feel. How you think and feel impacts and is impacted by chemical messengers. This works in the reverse direction as well. If you change your state, or how you think, your body will change in relation.

Of course, this applies to all areas of life. Alpha or dominant behavior includes having or taking control of your life in many different ways. This is important. Being dominant doesn't mean being an asshole, but it certainly means not being a wuss.

When I advise a positive attitude, it's not some "Pollyannaish" idea, but instead about self-responsibility. Take control of your own life. Only you can do it. If you leave things up to others that means you're not being an alpha. If you blame external circumstances for your woes than you have abdicated control. Once again, this isn't about being a dick.

It's about being confident and courageous. While high T levels help you to do this, the other way around works just as well. Higher testosterone will give you more confidence. And being more confident will fuel higher testosterone.

In one study that looked at the levels of testosterone and how dominant behavior was done they said (emphasis added), "In men, high levels of endogenous testosterone (T) seem to encourage behavior intended to dominate--to enhance one's status over--other people...**T not only affects behavior but also responds to it.** The act of competing for dominant status affects male T levels in two ways. First, T rises in the face of a challenge, as if it were an anticipatory response to impending competition. Second, after the competition, T rises in winners and declines in losers. Thus, there is a reciprocity between T and dominance behavior, each affecting the other...We contrast a reciprocal model, in which **T level is variable, acting as both a cause and effect of behavior**, with a basal model, in which T level is assumed to be a persistent trait that influences behavior."

So if you act like an "alpha" you'll increase your testosterone. And if you have higher testosterone you'll act like an "alpha". It works both ways. This is a critical distinction. But we're not done.

We've begun to explore the "meaning" of testosterone. If we look at the benefits of it, and the drawbacks of its deficiency, we can see some commonalities. Here are three areas that most men would agree are important.

1. Sexuality
2. Athleticism
3. Success (testosterone is sometimes referred to as the "success hormone")

While these might seem like three vastly different things, there is a common element behind them all. It's that masculine, driving, yang type of energy. When I first got into tonic herbalism I realized that herbs that were good for sex were also good for athletes and vice versa. It's because of this common theme behind them. And it extends beyond that.

All athleticism is harnessing that same energy. Most sports involve a ball, and many a stick or bat, which needs to enter a goal, and it's a man's job to get it there. Are you getting it yet?

Even war and violence has its basis in this same symbolism. Many weapons are noted to have phallic shapes which are then inserted like a sword or shooting the bullet from a gun into the enemy.

I've even heard money described as "financial testosterone". It's commonly used as a measure of success, even if it's not the best measure, it certainly is one measure. The drive to make money and build business is much the same.

So let's **penetrate harder** into the meaning of testosterone. Did you catch what I just said? That sexual reference explains much of it.

The world is often described as a duality. There's yin and yang. The feminine and the masculine. The yin, female energy is receptive. The yang, masculine energy is expansive, exploding, going outward.

Excuse me, if I get crude for a moment. It's necessary to drive this part home. In sex a man is inserting his cock into the woman. (Even among homosexuals, there is always a masculine/feminine dynamic going on.) That's yang into yin.

A man aiming at success is "**fucking the world**". He is using that same energy to create and manifest something he desires. It's **pro-creation** aimed in a different way.

Kim Anami, a holistic sex and relationship coach, and self-proclaimed vaginal kung-fu expert, teaches that many problems around impotence are not really physiological. Instead your "little man" acts like you, the "big man," in many ways. Thus if a man is being impotent in the outside world, it often is reflected to him in the bedroom. As we're talking about psychology this can become played out in various subtle ways.

This is the idea behind "Sexual Transmutation," which the author of *Think and Grow Rich*, Napoleon Hill talked about. His research showed that most men do not become successful in business until later in life, their 40's, 50's and beyond. His reasoning was that at a younger age they're too concerned with sex itself. He describes sex as an emotion, which is energy in motion. But beyond a certain age these men learn to direct this energy elsewhere.

There are some powerful practices that can be built around this. If you look as the energetic traditions, the chakra system corresponds directly to endocrine glands. The microcosmic orbit runs through all these areas. Various qi gong practices often have a sexual basis too. You are transmuting this energy from one area into another. These practices can very much influence the physiology of the glands that produce hormones from the pituitary to the testes and more. Even without this practice though, the idea alone here shows the meaning.

We can look more directly at the male genitals for more symbolism. As described by Dr. Carruthers, "The testis has to pluck up the courage to make a small step outside the body into the colder scrotum and testosterone drives it to do so."

The testicles, which are formed from the same tissue as ovaries in females, descend from inside the body out. The testes not descending, as sometimes happens, can become an issue with health ramifications. Note how he uses the word "courage" to describe this action. The balls, being extremely sensitive, hang out there, because of their need for a colder temperature than being inside the body would provide.

They just hang out there confidently like anything that manufactures testosterone would!

Although eunuchs are not common now, they use to be, because cutting off the balls would get rid of a man's sexual desire and the lust for power.

Castration is still used in animals to fatten them up and tenderize the meat. Castration is also used to domesticate wild animals. Cut the balls off and they become less tough and less wild. There's also such a thing as chemical castration. Instead of physically removing the balls, chemicals can be used to shut them down completely. As we'll discuss later, this is happening on a minor level everywhere with estrogen mimics.

Once again physical castration is very rare amongst humans these days (thankfully). But there is all kinds of psychological castration that can occur. This can be inflicted by others, if you allow them to do so. Probably even worse is that many people inflict this upon themselves.

Does your job or your boss leave you without balls? Does your wife or girlfriend carry them around in her purse? If so, is there any wonder why you don't have optimal testosterone? A man must own his balls if he has any hope of great hormone production throughout life.

This starts with the right attitude. The attitude then begins to direct your thoughts and your behaviors.

The balls also manufacture sperm. Over a lifetime a man will produce 525 billion sperm cells. Each ejaculate contains roughly 40 million to 1.2 billion of them. Why so much? Not all of them are made to fertilize the egg though. They're made to compete with one another as well as some are specialized to fight off other men's sperm. Leave it to men to produce far more than what is needed, and to be prepared for war!

Then we can talk about the penis. To do its procreative function it must stand tall and firm. This leads us into the next section…

Free Testing for Hormone Health

Every man knows what morning wood is. Cast your mind back to your teenage years and just how hard and frequently it happened. (Even in math class…)

Now you're probably older. Testosterone and other male androgens drop naturally as you age, though this may not be because of age itself but other factors compounded over time. With that drop you may notice another drop…

And here's the big idea of this section. **Morning wood is linked to testosterone.** When we dive into the detail we'll show you how.

But for now, understand that your morning wood, can be used as a leading indicator for how healthy your testosterone and other hormones are. Thus you can look at and feel how you're doing.

The technical term for morning wood is nocturnal penile tumescence (NPT). Nocturnal meaning night, penile meaning penis, and tumescence meaning the quality or state of being swollen. (I don't really think of it as swollen dick when I wake up, but that's the technical definition.)

Other common names include "morning glory," "pitching a tent," and "raising the flag", though morning wood is the most common.

But perhaps we should start using the term "Morning Steel" as this conveys something stronger than wood. We'll get to why this statement of quality may be important in a bit.

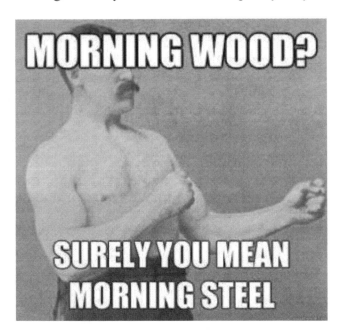

Morning wood is a natural part of the sleep cycle, occurring multiple times a night. There are several different stages of sleep which we cycle through several times in any given night. Many people know that the REM, or rapid eye movement, stage is accompanied by dreams. And it's also accompanied by wood.

The interesting thing is that your entire body is paralyzed during dreams, through neurotransmitters, except your erections. One of these is norepinephrine which causes vasoconstriction of penile blood vessels which prevents erections from occurring.

But during REM sleep, norepinephrine slows down specifically in a part of the brainstem known as the locus coeruleus. While this happens testosterone increases. Testosterone, which operates on a daily cycle, has its highest point of the day, in the early morning time. Testosterone appears to be a trigger for nitric oxide, which we'll talk more about later. But NO is what causes relaxation of the cavernosa which allows the blood to flow in and an erection to occur.

The locus coeruleus has several androgen receptors which your testosterone will activate. If you have sufficient free testosterone, with a few other factors likely at play too, then morning erections will occur.

One of the purposes of this happening is oxygenation of the tissues. Testosterone helps to repair and maintain functionality of the penis by triggering blood flow. So it operates as sort of a backup, in case you're not getting enough erections in your waking life. In addition, research urologists found that the increased blood flow helped to prevent excessive collagen from forming inside the erectile tissues.

It's basically use it or lose it. And without morning wood, some men would likely lose its functionality all together.

And here's a fun fact. Did you know that spontaneous erections occur even when in the womb? This is likely caused by the testosterone surges that helps a boy become a boy during the gestation, rather than a girl.

Another contributor to morning wood can be a full bladder. This is called a "reflex erection" as the full bladder stimulates a region of the spinal cord. The reason for this would be to prevent urination while sleeping. But it's important to note that this is not the only reason it happens as is sometimes believed.

However, this reflex poses its own problems, as any man with a massive erection can attest to. Going pee when you wake up in this state can pose a challenge. For that reason this handy infographic can help you out…

How To Pee With Morning Wood

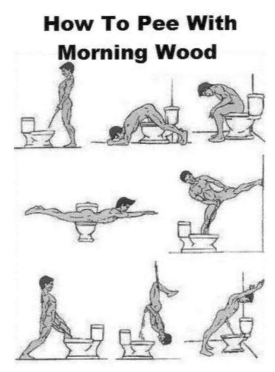

Otherwise known as the Manliest Form of Yoga

Analyzing Your Morning Wood (aka NPT Monitoring)

NPT monitoring (yes, that's a technical term) is often done in cases of erectile dysfunction to determine if there are physiological or psychological problems. In the early days something similar to postage stamps were placed around the dick in order to see if it got hard at night and broke the proliferation.

Nowadays, there's more scientific measurements, including a tool called a RigiScan. Recent research looked at several different factors including:

1. Tumescence activity unit
2. Rigidity activity unit values
3. Total erection number
4. Erection times

They even went so far as to distinguish between tip rigidity and base rigidity. To put this in laymen's terms its four different qualities.

1. Girth
2. Hardness
3. Number of Erections
4. Length of Erections

Now when I think of scientists measuring these things I get an image of them connecting my dick to various wires. I don't know if that's what they actually do, but it doesn't sound comfortable or like a fun procedure, unless I suppose if it was all hot, female scientists! I'm willing to bet that's a plot for a porn somewhere…

Anyway, we can look at these factors ourselves in order to better understand what our morning wood (or lack of it) is telling us, without needing any equipment.

Some of these are easier to measure than others. I don't expect you to take out a measuring tape so let's do away with girth. Besides, unless you have fine measuring skills this isn't likely to change too much from day to day.

Hardness or rigidity is going to be the strongest factor to look at. Instead of causing any sort of pain by seeing how hard your dick is to bend, I would simply rate in on a scale of 0 to 10 (with 0 being flaccid and 10 being strong as steel, and a 6 being you could probably use it for sex at this point but not ideal). So here you see why "Morning Steel" is our aim. Of course, this is subjective, but using a scale like this, will help you to know better over time.

The number of erections is something you can note down if you wake up multiple times in the night or morning and notice wood each time. In some cases the morning wood might wake you up. You could do the other measurements with each of these or just for your longest, hardest one.

The length of your erection is another important cue. Sometimes with morning wood you wake up with it and its gone almost right away. Other times it just won't seem to go down and lasts for many minutes. This is the kind where urinating becomes difficult. Once again, you don't need a stopwatch for this, just give a ballpark number. Does it go away fast, last about a minute, last about five, a half hour?

In addition to these factors you'll want to note down any special practices, diet changes, herbs or supplements you're taking that can be effecting these results.

With awareness you might even be able to tell the difference between a full bladder "reflex erection" and one that isn't caused by such. If you do any other sort of sleep tracking this is just a couple more data points to look at.

As an example, this morning I woke up with a hardness of about 8. Good solid wood, but not quite steel. This one lasted for probably over five minutes as I fell back to sleep. Later when I woke up I had some less hard, less long lasting ones, but there were multiple.

To help out I put together this handy chart on the next page. I recommend you print this out, multiple copies, and keep it by your bedside so that you can take down the information as it arises (pun intended).

Morning Wood Monitoring

www.SuperManHerbs.com

	SUNDAY	MONDAY	TUESDAY	WEDNESDAY	THURSDAY	FRIDAY	SATURDAY
Date:							
Sleep Time: Wake Time:							
Hardness (0-10)							
# of Erections							
Length of Erection							
Special Notes							

Testosterone and Morning Wood

Let's dive a bit deeper into the testosterone related action, as that's where this idea that morning wood is an important indicator of health comes from. I noticed this effect in myself and others long before I was able to find the research to back it up. But after a long search I was able to find these details.

As reported by Malcolm Carruthers, M.D., with emphasis added, "Although usually brief, these spontaneous morning erections are an important sign that the erection mechanism is working properly and has been primed by the testosterone surge which normally occurs around waking time. **Their loss in andropausal men is probably due to the overall decrease in free testosterone which I have found to be the key diagnostic feature** and by the reduction in the daily variation of testosterone levels with increasing age observed by me and reported by other researchers. **This view is supported by the fact that early morning erections are one of the earliest signs that potency has been restored by testosterone, and often happen within a week or two of starting treatment.**"

And here's another report, *The endocrinology of sexual arousal,* which a bit more technical, with emphasis added, "Nocturnal penile tumescence (NPT), the occurrence of spontaneous erections during rapid eye movement (REM) sleep, is relevant. The neurophysiological basis of NPT is still disputed, but one plausible explanation is that REM sleep is associated with a 'switching off' of the noradrenergic cells in the locus coeruleus (l.c.) (Parmeggiana & Morrison 1990) which, via their spinal projections, are probably associated with inhibitory tone in the penis. Thus, the reduction of inhibitory tone during REM permits what can be called 'excitatory tone' to be expressed as erection. **NPT is clearly impaired in hypogonadal men, and restored to normal with testosterone replacement. The l.c. has testosterone receptors (Parmeggiana & Morrison 1990), and this putative 'excitatory tone' can be regarded as testosterone dependent.** Carani et al. (1995) evaluated the effects of exogenous testosterone on NPT in eugonadal men. **Intramuscular testosterone enanthate had no effect on sleep parameters, and did not affect frequency, degree or duration of NPT, when assessed as penile circumference, but did increase, modestly but significantly, penile rigidity during NPT.**"

My personal experience, as well as many others, is it's not just rigidity that can be increased but much more. But I haven't been taking straight testosterone either. Perhaps that doesn't work as well as the things I'm about to share with you.

So with my personal experience and several others to back it up, this is why morning wood, especially the qualities of it described earlier, can be looked at as in indicator of testosterone in the body. There's also a second test…

The "Schwing" Feeling

Do you remember Wayne's World? It started as a Saturday Night Live skit with Mike Myers and Dana Carvey, as Wayne and Garth, and was made into two movies as well. They're most famous for their catch phrase "Schwing." They would say this when seeing or talking about hot women, and thrusting their hips into the air. This is described as the sound a sword makes as its being unsheathed.

If you're not familiar with it, here's a clip of Garth:
https://www.youtube.com/watch?v=2xTqUEhWYsI

While it refers to "popping a boner", I feel like there is actually more to it than this. Sure, the random boner that occurs at the sight of a woman, or for no reason at all, is a great sign of high T. But let's face it, that's not something we want to have all the time. If that's occurring than your T is probably doing great, or you're just a teenager.

To me, "schwing" implies more of an internal feeling. When you see an attractive woman, do you feel it in your balls instantly and automatically? Are you literally "attracted" to her like she is a source of gravity?

Some describe it as a tingle or tickle in their balls. For me, I feel the perineum flex. While I can consciously do this, it's the automatic reflex that occurs at those times. Or it's like a contraction in the prostate, similar as to what happens in orgasm.

This is why guys are said to think with their dicks, because this feeling of "I need to be inside that". Having this feeling means you're hormones are probably at least at good levels. According to Christopher Walker, who has made a study of testosterone like me, this level appears to be at least 300-400 ng/dL of total testosterone. Lower levels will likely see issues in libido and also potentially erections at various times, in the morning or otherwise. The evidence suggests that even higher levels then this to not however correlate with even stronger libido.

(It doesn't mean you have to act on it. Although research does show that men who are single or cheat tend to have higher testosterone than those in committed relationships. After all, we do have all that sperm. Unfortunately, sexless, or mostly sexless marriages, and relationships are both a cause and symptom of lack of testosterone but there are ways around this while be committed to a single person. This is a big topic, beyond the scope of this book. So this comes with a disclaimer. Increase your testosterone with caution.)

Going back to my lifelong testosterone insufficiency, until recently, I didn't feel this quite as significantly as I have in the past year alone. Previously, it was like I didn't understand "schwing" but now I get it, having done multiple things to get myself towards ideal testosterone levels, better than even when I was a teenager.

The important thing is to notice the feeling and then you can tell when you have it and when you don't. While blood and saliva testing is great, if you master the morning wood and schwing tests, you probably won't need it, at least as far as male hormone health is concerned. It's great for the details, so you can then laser focus on protocols, so let's move onto those.

Blood and Saliva Testing of Hormone Levels

If you have some of the symptoms of low testosterone it is useful to get tested. These will give you quantified numbers you can refer to which help in several ways. First of all, you can get tested later on and compare your numbers so you know whether what you're doing is working, besides by just feeling better.

Secondly, it can let you know which of the several hormonal interactions are going to be most important for you, thus you can better target what you do to change them. Do you have too much estrogen? If so, focus on detoxing that and limiting how much you get. Is your T low? Build that up. Is there too much SHBG? Work to lower that. And if you have multiple issues, which they tend to go together, do it all.

This chart describes the reference ranges for a "normal" healthy adult male with blood or serum testing. Note that many of these come with different measurements, and not every test uses the same format so be sure to double-check those and convert when needed.

Hormone	Normal Range
Testosterone	300 – 1000 ng/dL
Free T	3.5 – 17.9 ng/dL
DHT	31 – 193 ng/dL
DHT/T Ratio	0.052 – 0.33
SHBG	10.8 – 46.6 nmol/L
FSH	1.0 – 6.9 mlU/mL
LH	1.0 – 8.1 mlU/mL
E2	17.1 – 46.1 pg/mL
Cortisol (9AM)	140 – 700 nmol/L
Prolactin	2-15 ng/mL
Pregnenolone	13 – 208 ng/dL
Progesterone	0.27 – 0.9 ng/mL

Remember that these are average ranges. But we don't want to be average because the average health is declining, as these numbers were found out from average populations. It is best to be on the high side of the normal range for the androgens and lower in the range for the estrogens.

Also determining a reference range or optimal range is up for debate thus you may see different numbers in different places. Often any testing you get done will show a reference range and let you know if you're high or low compared to it. However we are all also individuals. Thus what is high for one person may not be for another.

Everyone likes to focus on total testosterone, but that may be the least useful of the numbers. The free testosterone as well as DHT are going to show much more whether you're hormonally optimized or not. What appears to get much worse with age typically is that free testosterone goes down as the result of increasing SHBG.

In addition, you'll want to look at your ratios between the hormones. While the amounts are important, the ratios will really determine your hormonal balance. Shoot for 80 to 120 times the total testosterone as estrogen. The ratio of E2 to T should be less than 1.

A less expensive and less invasive testing option is with the saliva. While you can't get all the different options that serum testing offers you can still get a fair amount. Because it is easier and cheaper to do, one of the useful benefits is that saliva can easily be taken at different points in the day to point out more acute differences. Since certain hormones can fluctuate significantly from hour to hour, like cortisol, this is useful.

It is important to note that with saliva testing only Free T is measure, not Total T. But if you get just this and estradiol you can have a fairly good picture of your sex hormone health, as this will take into consideration things like SHBG and aromatization.

Testosterone (pg/mL)	Estradiol (pg/mL)	T/E Ratio
Optimal Greater than 80 Good 55-80 Low 35-55 Deficient Less than 35	Elevated Greater than 2 Normal 1-2 Deficient Less than 1	Optimal Greater than 40 Normal 30-40 Low 20-30 Deficient Less than 20

Dr. Richard Cohen describes the T/E ratio as the "Masculine Ratio." People tend to think that with testing it is an exact science. But for the reasons already stated and much more this can be a tricky science at best. For much more information check out this interview I did with the doctor all about this subject.

https://supermanherbs.com/ep42-the-art-of-blood-and-saliva-testing-with-dr-rick-cohen/

Covering the Basics

We'll be diving deep into the details of working to optimize individual hormones as listed earlier. All of these advanced steps work, but if you don't cover the basics, you're probably not going to get the optimal results you desire.

What are the basics?

1. Drink plenty of high quality water

It is not just about quantity but also quality. Tap water can be one of the biggest sources of endocrine disrupting agents as will be discussed later. A high quality filter should be used at the very least. A good quality one that won't break the bank is available at http://legendarystrength.com/go/waterfilter/

Though an even better option is fresh spring water if it's available in an area around you.

Of course, the quantity is important too. Most people simply do not drink enough water. Dr. Batmanghelidj, in *Your Body's Many Cries for Water*, attributes all manner of disease, including pain, asthma, allergies, stress, depression, high blood pressure, obesity, arthritis and more to dehydration. He states you should treat thirst with medication and he's right.

I would recommend, at minimum, a half ounce of water per pound of bodyweight. Of course other factors like how much water is in the foods you eat, will play into this, but better to err on the side of too much, than too little, with water.

Think of it this way. NOTHING can be kept healthy in the human body under chronic dehydration. Hormones are just one of those issues so drink up. One observational study of wrestlers specifically looked at dehydration and noticed testosterone decreased and cortisol increased, compared to hydrated wrestlers.

For a deep dive into water see *Upgrade Your Water.*

2. Get quality and quantity of sleep

You cannot have high quality hormones without sleep. Just like water you can't have any aspect of health without it. Once again here it is a matter of both quantity and quality.

While some people can get by on less sleep, more so than others, it just plain isn't good for you to do so. Not everyone needs the recommended eight hours, some will be fine on seven, but really not less than that.

For hard charging athletes you need even more time to sleep, to aid in recovery. Melatonin is the hormone in "charge" of sleep, but also one of the body's strongest antioxidants. Growth hormone, then rises once you're asleep to help repair the body. Later, cortisol comes on the scene to help wake you up. You can bet with all of these, and more, that testosterone is affected.

Multiple studies have shown that LH and T decrease with lack of sleep, low quality sleep and fragmented sleep where waking up or abnormal breathing, like with sleep apnea, occurs.

Besides changing your life up to actually get the number of hours you need, some of the best tips for improving sleep quality are

- To black out your room from as much light as possible.
- Go to sleep at a regular time.
- Wind down away from any and all electronics, an hour before bed.
- Eliminate any sort of EMF fields in your bedroom and/or get grounded.
- Get direct sunlight in your eyes immediately when waking up or at sunrise if you're up before then.
- Use of select herbs or supplements to assist in sleep

Of course there is much more on this subject. For a complete run down on sleep check out *Upgrade Your Sleep*.

3. Get the right kind of exercise

This is covered in depth in the companion manual, *T-Boosting Workouts*.

4. Have a self-responsible, confident, positive mental outlook and be an "alpha"

This was covered in the previous sections. Do not underestimate how important your mental outlook is to testosterone. (And check how you're sitting or standing right now. Is it a high or low power pose?)

5. Eat organic and high-nutrient density food

Since nutrition is a hotly debated topic, what this means, especially when looking at hormone production will be discussed at length below.

If you cover these basics alone that's probably 90% of the battle, if you did them your whole life. But since most of us don't start nor always do this, we may have some tougher ground to make up.

The Macro-Nutrient Wars

As you'll come to see, the micro-nutrients that we consume, vitamins and minerals may be even more important than the macronutrients. That's because people tend to get "enough" macronutrients, whereas they can be chronically depleted of many micronutrients.

Still some focus on the three macronutrients is useful, when it comes to testosterone optimization. The three macronutrients are fat, carbohydrates and protein. Of course, not all fats are the same, not all carbs are the same, and not all protein is the same. Still, we'll use these three groupings to talk about what is important for hormone health.

If we want to distill it all down to something simple, it is you want a good amount of each, carbs, protein and fat, without having too much, for optimal hormone production.

Carbohydrates

Hot on the nutrition scene are many ketogenic diets. These diets basically eliminate carbs or move them down to very low levels. While these diets certainly have their place, and can be great short term for weight loss, cancer, diabetes, and even long term for a few select people it seems, they're not the best option for most.

When the body is devoid of carbohydrates, after some time it can switch over to an alternative fuel source besides glucose. Once ketosis is reached the body is burning ketones more for energy. (This is a simplification as glucose can still be used in some parts of the body, and even protein can be converted into glucose for the body to use.)

Working in the nutrition space I felt it was necessary to experiment with this. Although I only did it for a periods of less than two months, which some people would say isn't enough time to become fully keto-adapted, I had enough results that made me wish to stop.

First of all, my workouts were hit or miss. About half of them I had good energy for and the others I did not. While there is a fair amount of research showing the endurance athletes can become trained to use ketosis and then keep on enduring, that is not my sport. And you'll see that is not the training recommended for testosterone anyway. In my strength related endeavors, I suffered.

Secondly, my libido plummeted. It was sometimes there, but on many days I had no interested in sex. Thus, I had to call an end to this experiment.

Research shows that low carbohydrate diets can drive testosterone down. Part of this may be that low carbohydrate intake can elevate cortisol and other related hormones. SHBG also goes up with low carb intake. There are likely many reasons for this. One of which is that GnRH pulses less frequently wen there is less glucose available in the brain.

These researchers speculated that a higher carb/protein ratio was beneficial for testosterone.

Of course, eating too many carbohydrates can lead to all sorts of other issues, like insulin resistance. You'll hear this point brought up again and again, it's all about the quality of your food. Minimally processed carbs are generally going to be better than heavily processed carbs. This is regardless of whether they're simply or complex versions.

Compare a banana to high fructose corn syrup. Both simple sugars. Very different bodily reactions. Compare a piece of bread to a bowl of whole oats. Once again, very different.

In general, here is a general guideline of important, to least important food groups that contain carbs.

- Green leafy vegetables
- Low sugar fruits
- Starchy vegetables
- Fresh whole grains
- High sugar fruits

Grains can be problematic for many people leading some to swear off them completely. I personally eat gluten free the vast majority of the time and have gone one and off grain free. What I've been doing more recently is using raw unprocessed grains which I then soak and cook.

That being said it does look like there are a couple grains that may help testosterone production. Oats have earned a reputation for aiding in sexuality and hormone levels, sometimes attributed to the avenacosides in them, though I couldn't locate any primary research on this.

Sorghum, is not a well-known grain, but some research in vitro shows that it can increase DHT by increasing the 5-alpha-reductase enzyme.

Protein

Protein provides amino acids that the body uses for many different things, not just building up muscle. From the current research, it shows that protein is less responsible for testosterone than either fat or carbohydrates.

As before it is recommended to get as high quality protein sources as you can find. Meat, poultry and fish are all great sources. Eggs are another one. Dairy can be, if your body can tolerate it.

Then you can also get protein from nuts, seeds, as well as some in grains and beans. Fat almost always comes paired with protein in nature. Therefore, it stands to good reason that these should often be consumed together.

A good quality protein powders can make a fair substitute, but generally unless you're trying to pack on lots of muscle fast you don't need even close to a gram per pound of bodyweight. You probably don't even need half of that.

Research has shown that T levels were better in people that ate 10% protein compared to those that consumed 44% protein.

Fat

Fat is important, in that much animal fat is paired with cholesterol, the precursor of all the sex hormones. That will be discussed in some detail later. And beyond that, fat is important for a number of other reasons.

One of which is that every single cell membrane is made up with fat. Not only do we want to eat a sufficient quantity of fat, but also good quality fats. Whether animal, or plant based, this largely comes down to the quality of the fat, with a minimum of processing involved.

In the end you'll want a good supply of the three main types of fat, saturated fat, polyunsaturated fat (fish oil is the best here), and monounsaturated fat (olive oil being the classic example with a high amount). These can be further broken down into individual types of fatty acids.

What studies have found is that a higher amount of omega 6 to omega 3 ratio, which is common in the Standard American Diet is correlated with lower testosterone levels. Omega 6's are found in higher amounts of processed oils like corn, canola, soy, safflower, sunflower, etc. Omega 3's are found in most fish, grass-fed beef, and some nuts and seeds (besides walnuts, chia and flax, most are heavily skewed on having more omega 6's though).

Other research has found that higher levels of monounsaturated fats are good for testosterone. Beyond olives and olive oils, avocados are well known for these. The truth is all fats are mixes of these different types of fats, but the ratios are important. Many animal fats have lots of these fats in addition to saturated fats. Coconut is one source of saturated fat from the plant kingdom that is great to use in a variety of ways.

All in all, fat should probably make up 40+% of your diet, by calorie count not volume. Research has shown that this amount was superior to 20%. While we don't want to become ketogenic, nor go so high fat that there's no carbs, we do want to be what I call "fat-fuel adapted," meaning that your body knows how to burn fat for fuel and not just sugar. I am not saying that you need to count calories but that you should be aware of a good portion of your energy needs are coming from fat.

A good clue that you are fat-fuel adapted is that you'll be able to go hours without food (aka fast) for periods of time without feeling like you need food. Fasting can dramatically increase growth hormone, even when done for just short periods of time, aka intermittent fasting. Thus this will support putting you in an anabolic state.

So to some it all up, in the words of Sean Croxton, "Just eat real food." If you do that with fairly balanced amounts of carbs and fats, with a bit less protein, then chances are your testosterone is going to take care of itself. Organic high quality natural foods are going to place less of a toxic load on the body, while supplying more micronutrients and often phytochemicals that will support this goal. Then take some time to stop eating every once in a while.

Battling Testosterone's Enemies
The Anti-Androgens

More important than working on increasing testosterone itself is to combat all the many things, the anti-androgens, that can diminish testosterone's abilities, convert it to the opposite, or render it inert. We'll be covering the increasing aspect, but this area is where to start. That's because having good to optimal testosterone typically takes care of itself IF you do the things in this section. You are a man. You are meant to have good levels of testosterone. It's these things that stand in the way.

What's also important to note is that many of the recommendations for these problem areas, work on more than just one aspect. It's not like the drug-paradigm where a drug is supposed to do one thing, and one thing only. The truth is you can't effect just one thing, which is why drugs cause side effects. By forcing one issue, this in turn causes problems in other areas. So it's better to work holistically. Each of these goals in turn typically helps support the others.

Having the lab numbers from testing is going to best allow you to narrow in on what you do. That being said, I've ordered these steps in a way that I think would be appropriate for just about any man to follow. The first two especially are something we MUST do living in the environment we live in today.

1. Limit Endocrine Disruptors
2. Detox Endocrine Disruptors
3. Lower Cortisol
4. Lower Aromatase
5. Lower SHBG
6. Lower Prolactin

Step 1- Limit Endocrine Disruptors

One of the main reasons for the overall decline of testosterone in men through the years, regardless of age, is that our environment has become overly estrogenic in many different ways. This contributes to estrogen dominance. The extra bad part about that is that this sets up a vicious cycle. When estrogen is elevated, testosterone goes lower.

Sir Charles Dodds was the first to described xeno-estrogens in a paper from 1938 titled *'The Estrogenic Activity of Certain Synthetic Compounds.'* Yet it's only fairly recently that most of us have heard of these things. Sadly, in the 78+ years since they were first identified the problem has gotten far worse and much more pervasive.

I've used the term endocrine disruptor specifically for a reason. That means something that wreaks havoc on your endocrine system, i.e. hormones. Although many of these are estrogenic, that's not the only effect they can have.

Much of this have not been explored. One example is a metabolite of DDT, known as p.p.-DDE. This actually has little estrogenic activity, unlike DDT, but it is 15 times as anti-androgenic. It doesn't act like an estrogen but instead just stops androgens from working directly.

It's important to note that there is no widely available blood or saliva test for these chemicals in our body. They are unavoidable in modern day living, unless you live in a faraway cave, remote from any civilization. And the truth is they're probably in those remote locations because we've spread them around so much and they don't disappear easily. With test results you may see other hormones increase or decrease because of these, but it's typically not measured directly.

Here we'll focus on the different types of estrogens, which can be classed in a number of ways, depending on where they come from.

Xeno-estrogens are man-made and include pesticides, chemicals, plastics and more. Xeno-estrogens are probably the worst culprit of the groups because they're unnatural and that means the body often has trouble processing them. But they're not the only ones. Common sources include:

- Bovine Growth Hormone
- Tap water
- Laundry detergents
- Chemicals in sunscreens
- BPA, Phthalates and other chemicals found in most plastic
- PCB's
- Food coloring like Red 3 aka Erythrosine
- Parabens found in cosmetics and shampoos

- Pesticides like vinclozolin
- Insecticides like DDT, DDE, indane (banned in Europe but still in use in the USA), methoxychlor, etc.
- Fungicides like propiconazole (which happens to be so strong scientists have investigated it as male contraceptive!)

Sadly, we have over 90,000 man-made chemicals in our environment. Over 85% of these have never been tested for their effects on the human body. They're just assumed safe. Yet we know many chemicals do have deleterious effects.

But those are not the only problem. Phyto-estrogens are natural compounds found in nature. We're not the only one with sex hormones. And if we lived in a "natural" world these probably would not be a problem, but in combination with the other estrogens it might be best to avoid these completely, for anyone careful of their T, though there may be some cases for the proper use of them.

- Soy – Soy is touted for its benefits as a widely consumed component of Oriental diets. However they almost always eat it in fermented forms (miso, tempeh, natto) that break down estrogenic compounds in it. It is best to avoid processed soy foods like soy milk and tofu completely.
- Hops – Found in 99.99% of beers. The German Beer Purity Laws made it so hops were in every beer. This spread throughout the world. Before that time all kinds of herbs were used. Earlier beers using other herbs may have been androgen supporting! It was discovered that the women who collected hops for beers experience earlier menstrual periods. Also men suffered from reduced libido and feminization. More recently, research at the University of California found phytoestrogens in hops to bind to estrogen receptor sites. The common "beer gut" isn't just about the extra calories people get from drinking beer, but a symptom of excess estrogen.
- Flax seeds – Touted as a health food for its omega-3 content, this may lead to estrogen problems. A much better similar food is chia seeds. Although defatted flax seeds appear to help pull out excess estrogen from the body, so that may be useful in certain situations.
- Licorice root – A common harmonizing herb in many Chinese herbal formulas. Unfortunately it also has very strong estrogenic effects and can also inhibit progesterone.

Several of the female herbs, like damiana, shatavari, black cohosh, red clover and others have estrogenic activity, sometimes strongly. These effects may be useful in some cases, at least for women, but are probably best avoided by most men, or at least only used in limited fashion under proper supervision.

Once again, avoiding drinking a beer every once in a while because of the hops, when you're still painting chemicals onto your skin with body care products, is not the proper way to do it. Eliminate the worst offenders first.

Metallo-estrogens are a relatively unknown class. While many people in the field of health are aware of the problematic effects of heavy metal toxicity it is not well known that these metals contribute to estrogen dominance as well. This has been noted with lead, mercury, cadmium and vanadium. Heavy metal contaminated products include:

- Fish (farmed fish is even higher in heavy metals than wild caught)
- Most tap water supplies
- Household cleaning agents
- Cookware
- White Flour
- Deodorants
- Pharmaceuticals
- Pollution (simply breathing in major cities causes consumption of lead and other heavy metals)
- Mercury dental fillings
- Vaccines
- And much more

Myco-estrogens are toxins are from various fungi that contaminant many foods.

- Aflatoxins found in peanuts, cotton, corn and other grains.
- Ochratoxins found in beer, wine, coffee, and much more.
- Zearalenone found in corn, barley, wheat, oats and rice
- Most cheeses and coffee are full of various sorts.
- Black molds and other hidden dangers within your home.
- If you suffer from candida overgrowth your body may be producing excess estrogens from within.

How much does all this stuff really effect you? The bad news is that very small amounts of hormones can be quite potent. Here's an example. One common pharmaceutical drug is Premarin, which actually uses estrogen derived from horse's urine. When taken by people, portions of the drug are excreted out in waste. This gets into the environment while they still remain as active estrogenic compounds. Estradiol and the other estrogens can be measured coming out of many water treatment plants. In one case it was measured at a concentration of 14 parts per trillion. This is a very small amount, yet it was still enough to cause sexual problems in the fish downstream, including changing the sex of them.

Fortunately, these small amounts of estrogens won't make you a girl, but they certainly can cause problems. The documentary, *The Disappearing Male*, pointed out that fewer male children are being born, and boys have a higher chance of miscarriage.

This is why tap water was listed as an estrogenic contributor. Sadly, not everything is removed in the majority of water treatments.

Thus the first step, in boosting testosterone, is to limit the amount of estrogen mimics and other endocrine disruptors we get exposed to. In this day and age it is hard to completely eliminate them. But you can certainly do a lot to limit your exposure. Some of the simplest and biggest steps include:

1. Avoid conventional and heavily processed food and eat organic instead.
2. Avoid those foods that are phyto-estrogenic or may be contaminated with various estrogenic compounds.
3. Drink clean water.
4. Switch out synthetic skin care products for all natural. The best rule to follow is if you wouldn't eat it, it shouldn't go on your skin. Note that a lot of organic skin care products still aren't the best ever.
5. Avoid plastic as much as possible. Don't use it them to eat with or drink from plastic bottles.

It's also interesting to note that our food supply, at least the animal portion, is mostly female. Males are either castrated or treated with estrogen in order to make the meat tenderer.

Step 2 - Detox Endocrine Disruptors

Even if we limit estrogens and other chemicals we're still going to get some exposure. In addition the body produces its own endogenous estrogens. While some of these are absolutely needed for health, we want to make sure anything above that amount is properly removed from the body.

In addition to causing estrogen activity, many chemicals can increase aromatase activity or otherwise disrupt androgens.

Your liver is responsible for detoxing estrogens, among just about everything else, out of your body. This occurs in a couple different steps. First the estrogens must be metabolized. Secondly, they need to be removed from the body through elimination. Different nutrients help with different parts of this process.

First of all, eat your cruciferous vegetables. This includes kale, collard greens, cabbage, Brussels sprouts, kohlrabi, broccoli, cauliflower (which are all actually the same plant). Also included are horseradish, mustard greens, arugula, watercress, radish, daikon radish and more.

Maca, the Andean superfood, is also considered a cruciferous vegetable. While some people claim that maca increases testosterone, it seems to work more directly on increasing libido, while leaving the hormones as is.

Regarding these food also being goitrogenic, it's important to note that this doesn't appear to be a problem for most people. Also these goitrogens are reduced in cooking and an adequate supply of iodine will render this a moot point. It only seems to be the case with iodine deficiency. We'll discuss iodine as it is important for our goals here later. Still listen to your body to find if these food work for you.

These foods include indole-3-carbinol (I3C) and diindolylmethane (DIM) which specifically transfer bad estrogen into less destructive forms, and help to remove estrogen from the body. These indoles can increase the ratio of good to bad estrogens (2-hydroxy estrogens to 16-hydroxy estrogens, respectively). There is another similar compound, indole-3-acetate, which is found in these vegetables but isn't often included in the supplements.

Eating some cruciferous vegetables daily will do a lot for your health. I frequently have a large portion of them, always cooked, and usually steamed. Adding fat, like grass-fed butter or coconut oil to these, will improve the absorption of many nutrients.

Pomegranates and berries are also great estrogen fighting foods. They contain ellagic acid which helps to draw estrogens out of the body. Another useful compound is calcium-D-glucarate, which is a fiber that is found in most berries. A similar compound, glucaric acid is also available in some other fruits including oranges, apples, grapefruit, as well as cruciferous vegetables. It specifically supports phase II liver detoxification. It binds to metabolized estrogens and other toxins, eliminating them from the body so they're not reabsorbed.

Bad estrogens are typically those that are missing methyl groups. So if you eat foods or take supplements that provide methyl donors your body can detox out the estrogens. Methyl donors include B6, B12 (the methylcobalamin form), folic acid, choline, MSM, TMG, DMG, SAM-e and DMAE as well as some of the amino acids like methionine, cysteine, serine, glycine.

Some of these compounds are found in onions, garlic, goji berries, and notably, beets which are very high in TMG. TMG stands for trimethylglycine, the original betaine, discovered in beets. It has three methyl groups it can donate, meaning that beets may be the best option for this form of detox. Beets work great in juice and also are great steamed or baked.

Quercetin, as found in onions and garlic, is another estrogen fighter. So is the sesamin found in sesame seeds, which like DIM, can convert estrogens into better forms.

While you can take supplements here, like an I3C/DIM combo, I believe sufficient amounts can be gotten from foods if you make sure to eat them often. Here are my top picks in order:

- Cruciferous Vegetables
- Berries
- Beets and Beet Juice
- Pomegranates
- Onions and Garlic

Add these into your regular diet and your body will do much better at detoxing estrogens (and that's only some of the benefits these foods can bring). Really you can't go wrong with low sugar fruits and green leafy vegetables.

One of the other big benefits that you get, which you won't get from supplemental forms of these, is they all have good amounts of fiber. While fiber may not directly affect your testosterone levels we need fair amounts of it for many other functions.

Step 3 - Lower Cortisol

If you go back to one of the pictures earlier in this book showing the conversions of different hormones, from cholesterol all the way down to testosterone and beyond, you'll notice a whole section that was only briefly discussed. This is the corticoids, of which there are many, the most well-known being cortisol.

First of all, the stress hormones, cortisol, as well as the adrenal hormones, epinephrine and norepinephrine (also called adrenaline and noradrenaline) are all catabolic in nature. They work against anabolic nature of testosterone and other androgens. So they directly counteract some of the effects.

And the other piece is that pregnenolone, progesterone and its metabolite, instead of converting into androstenedione which later becomes testosterone, can be converted into the corticoids. They call this "pregnenolone steal".

These are stress hormones, and while we certainly need some of them to live and be healthy, too much will cause numerous problems. (A future volume in the *Upgrade Your Health* series will look more specifically at cortisol, adrenaline and all the other associated hormones.)

One of the problems, if you're under too much stress, is that the building blocks for the sex hormones are all being stolen in order to make extra cortisol. If they're being converted into cortisol than it cannot convert into testosterone. Numerous studies point to the interdependency of these two hormones.

Stress can take many shapes and forms. It's not bad by itself, unless it's more than you can handle. Thus lowering stress can come in many forms:

Changes in Mindset and Perception

A tiger chasing you down for food is stressful. That's why the body has this system, to help us get out of dangerous situations. But since we've gotten out of the food chain, we largely don't have life threatening acute dangers like this. Instead our stressors are chronic. It can be the bills, the kids, the fight with the loved one, the traffic and so on.

However, something that stresses us out is because we've made it so. If you're frantic because you're late for an appointment you can stress out all about it. Or you can relax and then your body and mind won't read the danger the same.

Simply changing how you view stress can be a big component to not getting trapped in its deleterious effects. The truth is we need stress to grow. It's about getting the right amounts and something that helps with that is simply in how we perceive it.

Meditation

One of the best methods for learning to take a more stress-free outlook is various forms of meditation. There are hundreds of types that you can do. There are even apps to help you to it. Lots of people have trouble getting into the habit of meditating, but know that just one minute can make a difference.

Breathing Exercises

Many types of meditation have a basis in focusing on the breath. By taking deeper breaths and focusing on doing so you can reach a relaxed state. There are lots of different methods and cadences for doing so. For much more, not just on meditative breathing, but all sorts of breath work check out *Upgrade Your Breath*.

Walking

I don't really think of walking as exercise. It's just a human movement we ought to do. It has many benefits and one of which is that it can be a great stress reliever, especially when you spend time with over people you care about walking at a leisurely pace.

Qi Gong and Tai Chi

These can bring the benefits of the previous three categories of meditation, breathing and slow movements all together in one. A recent study not yet published, coming out of Cal Poly showed that athletes that spent 15 minutes a day doing qi gong exercises, were better rested, had lower cortisol, and significantly improved in their workouts, over others who do not engage in qi gong.

Laughter

Once of the best ways to relieve stress is to laugh. Get social with people that you enjoy spending time with and make you laugh. Watch comedy shows, movies or stand-up. The saying "Laughter is the best medicine" certainly has some truth to it.

Avoiding Excessive Exercise

One of the big issues of exercising right for testosterone is avoiding doing too much. Too much can take many forms. Too much intensity. Too much volume. Too long. Too often. Exercise by its definition is a stressor. Once again, the issue is the amount. Anyone of these can become too much and then contribute to the problem rather than helping it. Once again, see the companion manual, *T-Boosting Workouts*, for more detail.

Foods

Of course, the right food choices, as have been detailed as well, can cut down on dietary forms of stress too. If your body doesn't like something, like a food allergy to dairy, gluten, eggs, or anything else, even though you many not notice symptoms, it will stress the body.

There's also the mental side of things. Don't get so stressed out on your food choices that everything isn't perfect. I find it's best to follow an 80/20 or 90/10 rule with food. Eat high quality most of the time then allow yourself to eat what you want the rest. Still overtime, you'll want even your "cheat" food to be higher quality. After all you can still have cakes, cookies and pizza that is made with natural ingredients rather than loaded with chemicals.

The important thing is not to beat yourself up about what you eat. This truly can cause more harm than the food.

Adaptogens

Several herbs, known as adaptogens, are said to help the body adapt better to stress and have effects on cortisol. These includes rhodiola, eleuthero, schisandra, cordyceps, licorice, and others such as found in *Spartan Formula* at https://supermanherbs.com/spartan-formula/

Another thing you may want to be careful with is caffeine, especially coffee. I think coffee can be great, but caffeine does directly stimulate the adrenals to release cortisol. If you're suffering from high cortisol it would be best to skip the caffeine for a period of time.

Vitamin C, in addition to supporting the immune system and many other functions, helps the body to clear cortisol, as well as blunt it from spiking too high.

There are many other methods of working with stress and cortisol. But if you do just a few of these basics, along with everything else covered your cortisol will likely be in control. A further benefit of cortisol regulation is better sleep which then will assist in the other hormones too.

Step 4 – Lower Aromatase

Our next step is to limit the amount of testosterone that is being converted into estrogen. Before we get into that there's two important things to note.

First of all, excess body fat creates more aromatase, as the enzyme is created by your body in white adipose tissue. Contrary to old scientific opinion, fat is not inert but seems to be active endocrine tissue. This means if you want to optimize your testosterone, if you're overweight, you're going to have to lose that fat.

On that note, doing all the steps as recommended here, with the diet and strength training especially, will help you naturally arrive at that end. This isn't meant to be a diet, but when you trade out processed foods for more natural ones you can't help but to return to a more natural size.

Secondly, the worse off you are, the worse off you are. There's a feedback loop that as testosterone levels go down, aromatase activity increases creating a vicious cycle.

Aromatase activity is known to increase with age, obesity, insulin, alcohol, LH, FSH. With the LH and FSH, it's because it is involved in the feedback cycle so that not too much testosterone is created.

Aromatase is also inhibited by prolactin, but for other reasons discussed later we may want to lower that hormone, if it's excessive.

It's not just fat tissue that upregulates aromatase. Inflammation appears to be another issue. Thus, higher intakes of omega-6 fatty acids, promotes this estrogenic activity.

There are drugs, like Arimidex, designed as aromatase inhibitors, but also many natural sources which we'll cover here.

Apigenin, and other similar compounds, can be found in some fruits and vegetables including parsley, artichokes, celery, cilantro, basil, apples, cherries, mangosteen and grapes. Herbs containing apigenin include dandelion root, chamomile, bacopa, oregano, tarragon, and rose hips.

Celery, with its high luteolin content, works to inhibit aromatase. Celery also contains androsterone, the pheromone, secreted in sweat and byproduct of testosterone metabolism, which has been shown to cause attraction in women.

It's shown that numerous phytoestrogens actually have aromatase inhibiting activity. These were previously discussed, but I think just by the fact that they have some estrogenic activity doesn't mean they're all bad.

Some other aromatase fighting compounds include various polyphenols found in many foods like:

- Resveratrol from red wine
- Curcumin in turmeric
- ECGC from tea
- Oleuropein, found in olive oil
- Grape seed extract
- Agaricus bisporus, the common white button mushroom
- DIM, previously covered for detoxing estrogens, is also an aromatase blocker
- Nettle root
- Tongkat ali

So here we find, there's fewer regular foods that have these effects, and instead we'll turn more toward herbal allies. Note that several of these include culinary herbs like basil, parsley, oregano, turmeric and more. Why don't you try adding these to some of your meals, including to the cruciferous vegetables or beets from the previous step? And then taking some supplemental herbs will further help. Nettle root and tongkat ali will be discussed in more detail in the following sections.

None of these are going to work on the same level as a drug like Arimidex. Nor do we really want it too. But if we get a wide complement of some of these aromatase inhibitors in our natural diet, if we're doing all the other steps it can be sufficient.

If you're overweight, work on losing the weight, and eat these foods and herbs. If you're not overweight, just eat these foods and herbs.

Zinc is also one of the best aromatase inhibitors. We'll specifically address this critical mineral later.

Step 5 - Lower SHBG

Here is another step that might not be the most important, unless you find from testing you have high SHBG. I personally have had this be the case in a couple of the blood tests I've done, so it's an area I've spent a little additional time on. It's also something that naturally goes up with age.

Your liver controls how much SHBG and albumin is circulating in your body. Remember that albumin only weakly links to testosterone and other hormones so it isn't much of a concern. It's SHBG that takes largely them out of play. While it also binds to estrogens, it prefers DHT and T.

SHBG decreases with higher levels of insulin, growth hormone, IGF-1, androgens and PRL. High estrogen and T4 causes it to increase.

SHBG appears to be the reason that low carb diets have been linked to lowering testosterone. As you see above, higher insulin, decreases SHBG. If you're not using much insulin, which certainly you want to be avoided in excess, too little may be a problem too.

Cast your mind back ancestrally. In the spring and summer seasons many more carbohydrate food sources would be available, at least in most areas. These could be used to store body fat for the coming winter, as well as unleash that spring energy, in the form of more testosterone.

While there are certainly uses for ketogenic diets, and they seem to work fine for some long term, my experience with it did see a pretty substantial decrease in libido, meaning it probably ended up lowering testosterone, and possibly through the action of SHBG.

But carbs aren't the only important macronutrient. In one study over 100 grams of fat per day decreased SHBG. This was followed by putting the same people onto a low fat diet where their T went down and SHBG went up.

Alcohol also appears to raise SHBG. This is likely because the liver produces SHBG and drinking too often may impair this in some way. Lay off the alcohol and support your liver in a number of ways to help normalize SHBG.

Doing a fast every once in a while, which not only allows your digestive tract to rest, but allows the liver, which typically works all the time, some extra time to process and catch up on its work.

So besides eating sufficient fat and carbs, without going to too many of them, and not going excessive on alcohol what can you do?

Several vitamins and minerals including boron, vitamin D, magnesium, EPA/DHA, and zinc appear to have action on lowering SHBG. Looking at that list it covers many things that most people are deficient in. So it rising SHBG any wonder? Each of these are discussed more later.

I have a theory that aging people in Western societies are seeing such higher amounts of SHBG because of the excess of estrogenic chemicals. It's possible that the human body is producing more SHBG to try to bind to these and transport them around. It's just that this has a higher affinity for the androgens. Just a theory though, as I haven't seen evidence to back this idea up specifically. If this is the case, then the previous steps all will help here too.

As for herbal supplements, the main player here is nettle root. It has several compounds inside, and it seems the lignans have the ability to bind to SHBG. Nettle root also happens to be an aromatase inhibitor, making it one of the top hormonal assistants for men, working in ways besides increasing testosterone directly or indirectly.

You can find more about nettle root and pick up a bag at https://supermanherbs.com/nettle-root/

However, nettle root can also reduce DHT as well, by reducing 5-alpha reductase activity which creates DHT from testosterone. More about that later. On the flip side it certainly stops SHBG from binding to DHT leaving more of it free. So you'll have to see how it works for you.

Note also that it is the root of the stinging nettle plant. The leaves, seeds and other parts of this plant are used differently, although it's a powerfully medicinal plant overall.

To support your liver you can use burdock, dandelion root, schisandra and many other herbs.

Step 6 - Lower Prolactin

If your prolactin is high you may want to work on lowering this, as high prolactin levels are linked to low libido and testosterone, in addition to gynecomastia, better known as man boobs. That being said, not everyone will need to work on this hormone pathway.

You don't want it too low though. As we've seen higher prolactin was also associated with lower levels of aromatase and SHBG. That's why this is the final piece in this series, that may be important for some, but not for others.

The interesting thing about prolactin is that it appears to work opposite or antagonistic to the neurotransmitter dopamine in many ways. Higher dopamine levels are linked to higher testosterone synthesis and growth hormone secretion through its effects on LH, through GnRH.

As a rich source of L-dopa, the precursor to dopamine, Mucuna pruriens, may help to suppress prolactin, leading to some of its hormonal boosting effects. In a study in India with normal healthy and fertile men, mucuna increased LH by 23% and total testosterone by 27%. Prolactin decreased by 19%. In infertile men these changes were even bigger. My guess is that there is more hormonal action to mucuna then is known or hypothesized now. Find out more at https://supermanherbs.com/mucuna/

But mucuna does not work for every person. Some people feel their mood is altered in non-beneficial ways. Others experience nausea when taking it. Some research has had people become hyper-sexual by it. So by all means try it and see if it works for you, but you don't have to take it.

Dopamine is used as part of our reward drive. It's not released when we get a reward but more so in anticipation of a reward. Thus it can also be problematic with addictions. A healthy way to increase dopamine is through novelty, which is doing new things.

Stress also increases prolactin, giving you another reason to avoid excessive amounts. Good quality sleep will also help regulate this hormone.

Gluten, found in many grains, is also linked to increasing prolactin. Some other nutrients and herbs that have been shown to work on lowering prolactin include ashwagandha, zinc and vitamin B6.

Increasing Testosterone and Its Allies

Now that we've cut down and battled the anti-androgens, the dark side of male hormone health, it's time to focus on the light side, specifically working with testosterone and its various allies.

Understand that fighting the anti-androgens is probably more than half of the battle. If you take care of those things, then chances are you'll see a big boost in your health and performance.

And when you add in these steps it will do even more. Remember that many of these hormones can get trapped in vicious cycles, meaning the worse off you are the harder it becomes. This also means you can get stuck in the opposite, in virtuous cycles, where the better off you are, the easier it is to stay that way.

You'll notice I've been using a war metaphor. One way to think about this is if you had a tiny army going against a big army it's going to take some time to really see results. And you'll have to be smart about it. But if you have a big army, it's pretty easy to stay in control, as long as you continue to do mostly the right things.

Some of these steps include specific nutrients, which are necessary building blocks. From there we turn our focus to the cells themselves then the specific hormones and what we can do to increase them.

1. Cholesterol
2. Micronutrients
   a) Zinc
   b) Iodine
   c) Boron
   d) Fat Soluble Vitamins
   e) Choline
   f) Other Important Vitamins and Minerals
3. Sunshine and Vitamin D
4. Cell Receptor Health
5. LH and Other T Precursors
6. Testosterone
7. DHT

Step 1 – Cholesterol

Cholesterol is the building block for ALL of the sex hormones. Therefore it is of the utmost importance.

Yet, so many people have become scared of cholesterol because of its so-called impacts on heart disease. But this is largely not true. There are several books like *The Great Cholesterol Myth* by Dr. Stephen Sinatra and *Cholesterol Clarity* by Jimmy Moore that cover this in far better detail than I could do justice with here in a short amount of space. High cholesterol levels are actually trying to protect your body from damages and thus are a lagging indicator of problems.

Statins, the type of drug to lower cholesterol, are probably one of the worst drugs for your sex hormones because it does lower cholesterol, even if it doesn't lower the chance of heart attacks. If you're on these, I'd work with your doctor to get healthier so that you can possibly come off of them.

Suffice to say, you should eat cholesterol. This forms the building blocks for testosterone, all other androgens, as well as for the estrogens, corticoids and others as well. It's needed for every sex hormone.

The human body can create its own from scratch in amounts up to 1000 mg per day. For comparison purposes a large egg has about 187 mg. We'll talk more about eggs in a second.

As with many bodily processes it takes up some energy and resources. The liver makes most of it, though it can also be synthesized in the intestines, adrenals and reproductive organs. Why not save those resources, and the effort of the liver, since it has so much else to do, and just eat a fair amount of it?

Animal fat, as we've already talked about, is the source of cholesterol. Eggs, cheese, milk, beef, pork, poultry, fish, shrimp and more have it. Human breast milk is also a rich source. (Not saying you should drink this, it just proves the importance in growing healthy babies, and otherwise it wouldn't be in there.)

Cholesterol is not found in plant foods. This is the reason that many vegetarians and, more so with vegans, can have lower testosterone levels then their omnivorous brethren. I'm not saying you can't have good testosterone levels on these diets, but it is certainly tougher to do for this reason alone.

Specifically eating cholesterol appears to increase the HDL in the body, which is often called the good cholesterol.

I want to take a moment to talk about how great eggs are. The white part is a complete protein. This is actually better cooked, as raw it has some inhibitors in it, though it's still okay to eat. Fear of raw eggs and salmonella is overblown. If you get good quality eggs, rather than factory farmed, you're pretty safe. If you're still worried soak it in a pot of water. If any bubbles come out of the egg, that means the seal has been breached and it could possibly be contaminated. Otherwise it is safe.

But the real nutrition of an egg is in the yolk. This is best raw, as there are some delicate components. But lightly cooked is fine. What is best is to not oxidize the cholesterol as that can make it tougher for the body to use. Soft poached, soft boiled, sunny side up, or over easy are the best options. Scrambled or any version of a hard yolk is still okay, just not quite as optimal.

Along with the cholesterol you'll get plenty of other nutrients. Here quality certainly matters. The best eggs are going to be from pasture raised chickens. In these you'll find significantly more minerals and fat soluble vitamins, as well as choline. Many of these are explored in the next step.

Step 2 - Micronutrients

Nutrition is actually much more about the micro-nutrients, then the macro-nutrients that everyone pays attention to. If you don't have a full complement of micronutrients you can kiss your testosterone production goodbye.

Some of these are dramatically more important than others and are addressed directly below. We've seen many of these already mentioned in their roles in fighting various anti-androgens and they do even more than that.

A) Zinc

Our first micronutrient of critical importance is zinc. Zinc has many functions in the body including several hormonal ones. Zinc is used in the conversion of androstenedione into testosterone, and vice versa. It is likely a co-factor in several other androgen conversion steps as well.

Tons of studies have shown that in testosterone deficient men, supplementing with zinc, increases testosterone. It doesn't boost it by itself, but it is a required component in order to maintain healthy and optimal levels.

In addition zinc is a powerful aromatase inhibitor and lowers both SHBG and prolactin. Basically it's needed in EVERY component of testosterone health.

Zinc is also needed for sexual potency. Each ejaculate contains about 5 mg of zinc as it's a component in both the semen and the seminal fluid. As the RDA is only 11mg for adult males, some people will need to be sure to get more daily, just for this reason alone!

Good sources of zinc include shellfish, beef, lamb, liver and pork. Zinc in animal sources is the most bioavailable.

One of the classic highest zinc foods are oysters. In fact it is magnitudes higher than other foods. The great lover Casanova was said to consume many oysters every single day. Although there is variation, due to size and other factors, a single oyster typically has over 5mg of zinc. I'm fortunate to live near the ocean and can get fresh oysters regularly, but even if you can't you can often find smoked oysters canned. I like to use these as a snack, including taking some with me when travelling.

Nuts and legumes are also fairly high in zinc. One of the best recommended sources of zinc is pumpkin seeds. The problem here is that phytic acid, found in these as well as grains, inhibits zinc absorption. This can be remedied by soaking and/or sprouting nuts, seeds, legumes and grain before use. Cashews are also a decent source.

One thing to be aware of is that for both plants and animals the amount of zinc they'll contain depends on what is available in their food supply which all goes down to the soil.

In the 1930's farmers went in front of Congress to tell them the soil was basically depleted of this mineral, among others. That means any commercially grown crops, and also probably most organic food as well, won't have as much zinc as may be necessary. If it was bad then, it's even worse now!

In addition, high levels of estrogen disrupt zinc uptake in the intestines, while androgens support its uptake. Here's another place where you can get caught in a vicious cycle.

Another strike against alcohol is that it can impair zinc absorption too.

Unfortunately, there is a good chance you will not be getting sufficient amounts of zinc from your diet alone unless you're very particular and smart about it. It is commonly told that white marks in your fingernails are a sign of zinc deficiency. Pretty much my entire life I've had these marks but here is a picture from recently. There's still some tiny specks but nothing like what it used to be.

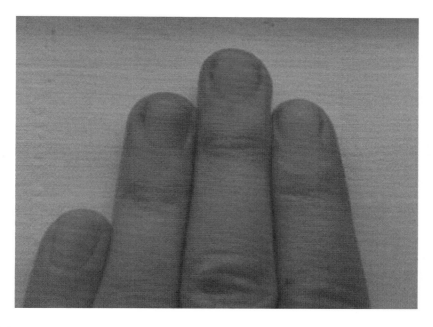

Because of the lack of it in a lot of food, and that we need a good amount, it may be worth supplementing with zinc. The best forms of isolated zinc supplements are zinc gluconate, zinc acetate, zinc citrate and zinc orotate which is shown to have the best absorption.

If you're making up for a deficiency of zinc you may want to supplement with 25mg up to even 100 mg per day for a period of time.

For me I try to get it from diet directly. In addition to eat oysters whenever possible, I eat a fair amount of meat, including organs. There are a few herbs that have fair amounts of zinc, but nothing I've found with super amounts.

B) Iodine

Iodine is commonly thought of as the important mineral for the thyroid. While it is, the fact is that iodine is used in every single one of your cells. And most people are deficient in it. Iodine is also important in modulating estrogen, and it has effects on T, FSH, LH, cortisol and insulin. It is definitely a hormonal mineral.

One thing iodine does is take the place and push out the toxic halides that your body has absorbed including fluoride, chlorine (both found in many municipal water supplies) and bromine (included in white flour, Gatorade and many other foods). PCB's are one particular threat. These toxins contribute to hormonal problems. They're attracted to the thyroid as well as the Leydig cells and block, even calcify, androgen receptors.

Thus iodine is an androgen ally that directly works against some potent anti-androgens. For that reason it's important to pay attention to this mineral specifically.

Iodine is hard to get from our diet these days. Besides, the RDA is quite low according to several doctors and others in the health field. Because of our environment, most people will need supplemental iodine to support an optimal level. An ideal amount may be higher, though there is debate as to how much is too much. Some research with rats showed that too much could cause damage to the testes.

While you can get small amounts from iodized salt, this salt is best avoided for other reasons as it is stripped of all other minerals, and instead is full of chemical agents. Unfortunately, most sea or rock salts don't have much iodine.

One fair source is seaweeds. Some seaweeds have way more than others. Bladderwrack, kelp and Irish moss are the highest. Wakame, alaria, dulse and all decent. But nori and sea lettuce are actually pretty low.

Fish like salmon, cod, tuna and sardines as well as shellfish like shrimp and scallops are decent sources. Eggs, with pastured eggs being much higher, and dairy can be too. Tiny amounts can be found in some fruits and vegetables.

With a supplement you often just need a couple drops to get a therapeutic dose. There are both iodine and iodide forms. Lugol's solution is a mixture of the two and is a good place to start.

We'll revisit iodine again when we talk specifically about cell receptor health.

C) Boron

Boron is an interesting mineral in that its elemental form isn't found on earth but instead in meteorites. It is a trace mineral, of which only small amounts are needed. However, recent research points to it being important for hormonal health, among other effects.

It appears to increase testosterone levels, modulate estrogen, plays a role in Vitamin D metabolism, improve muscle coordination, build strong bones and much more. One study even found specific increases in free testosterone, DHT and a decrease in SHBG).

Animal research points to boron assisting in the utilization of vitamin D. This in turn undoubtedly has an impact on the other hormones, since it is a hormone precursor. It is probably a good idea to make sure you have sufficient boron along with any supplemental vitamin D to assist its use.

The RDI is not established for this trace mineral. A tolerable upper limit appears to be 20 mg per day before side effects are seen. The US National Institutes of Health state that normal boron intake is 2.1-4.3 mg/day, though some people seem to get much less, often less than 1 mg/day, which does appear to cause deficiency.

I would say an optimal amount is somewhere in the 3-10 mg/day range. Therapeutic doses used in some of the treatments mentioned above are typically between 1 and 6 mg per day and this is taken as supplementation in addition to what is acquired in the diet.

Boron is mostly found in non-citrus fruit and vegetable sources. In general plant sources tend to be better than animal sources. Brazil nuts, almonds, hazel nuts, cashews, peanuts, walnuts are all good sources.

Raisins top the list at 4.51 mg/100 grams. Other dried fruits like apricots, prunes and dates are also decent. Of foods that you're more likely to eat a lot of, per 100 grams, avocado has 2.06 mg, kidney beans has 1.4 mg, brazil nuts 1.72 mg. Coffee and wine also appear to be decent sources.

Ionic boron also seems to work well as a supplement. Many other forms are used including boron citrate, boron glycinate, boron aspartate, calcium borogluconate and others. With minimal research it's hard to judge what the best option is.

Supplemental amounts of 3-10 mg is what has been used in most of the studies showing many of the different benefits. This dosage appears to be completely safe.

D) Choline

Choline is sometimes called vitamin B4, but is better known simply as choline. It can be created in the human body, but not in sufficient amounts for optimal health, and thus must be attained through diet.

It has multiple functions within the body. The first one is the structural integrity of cell membranes, as well as in their signaling mechanisms. This makes it important for the cell receptor health soon to be covered.

It is used in the production of the major neurotransmitter acetylcholine and is also converted into trimethylglycine. TMG is important for detoxing the body, including of estrogens, with its methyl groups as was covered before.

The recommended daily dose for men is 550mg/day. Eggs are a great source of choline with about 147mg per large egg. Liver is one of the best sources with 473mg per five ounces. Some other great sources are broccoli, cauliflower, spinach, cod, chicken, quinoa and amaranth.

E) Fat Soluble Vitamins

We've seen the important of fat. We've seen the importance of cholesterol. Along with those we typically get a dose of fat soluble vitamins. We'll be addressing vitamin D separately because getting it from diet is not the best method. That leaves A, E and K.

One thing I've come to realize is that many minerals and vitamins are concentrated in animal based products, while different minerals and vitamins are concentrated in plant based products. Here you find many more of the fat soluble vitamins in animal products.

Vitamin A has a few different forms. The preformed fat soluble form is retinol. The more common plant form is beta-carotene. The latter can be converted, but it is a process that is done so at a small percentage within the body.

Some vitamin A is actually stored in the testicles showing that it has a role there. In an interesting study looking at twins, it was found that those with vitamin A deficiency had lower testosterone levels.

Vitamin E comes in many different forms. Some research came out saying that people who supplemented with vitamin E were less healthy than people that didn't. But this was because most vitamin E supplements only contained one of at least eight forms. You need both tocotrienols and tocopherols.

Vitamin E is a potent antioxidant among many other functions. Some research has shown that deficiency in this impairs not only testosterone but LH and FSH as well.

Vitamin K use to be known just for the function of helping the blood clot. We now know that it does far more. As with other vitamins there are several forms you want, both K1, found more in plant foods, and K2 found more in animal foods. In a rat study supplementing with K2 saw a 70% increase in blood levels of testosterone.

F) Other Vitamins and Minerals

The B-vitamins don't seem to directly play a role in the sex hormones, though we saw B6 help with SHBG. Nor does vitamin C, but as we saw that is important for cortisol.

Still, basically every vitamin is going to be needed for optimal hormone health. So are minerals.

Magnesium is a nutrient that it is estimated about 90% of the US population is deficient in. It plays a role in over 300 different bodily processes. One study did find higher levels of free testosterone with magnesium supplementation.

Chromium plays an important role in insulin and blood sugar regulation. These are important for body fat and obesity, which as we've seen will ramp up aromatase and thus estrogen.

I could go on and on. And the truth is most of the trace minerals are not well studied for their various effects. In the end I'm willing to bet every nutrient can in turn be related back to testosterone. That's because the body works as a whole system, not a bunch of disparate parts.

So what do you do about it? The simplest solution is to make sure you are on a well-rounded multi-vitamin and mineral supplement. Unfortunately, they are not all created equal, not by a long shot. If you think you're getting covered by any of the popular one-a-day multivitamin, the truth is many of those may be doing more harm than good.

I'm all about getting what you need from real food. Yet I recognize that even eating the highest quality food and taking various herbs may still leave you with gaps when it comes to these nutrients. You'd have to be extremely careful and exact to get everything you really need for optimal functioning.

These days I feel my diet is pretty good and I could probably get away without taking this, but it took me years of working on my diet, getting it higher and higher quality, to get to this place.

If you are just starting to focus on your health, then basically you need something like this. Thus for many people the best bet is to make sure you have micronutrient insurance. For much more on this subject make sure to check out this interview with Jayson and Mira Calton, leaders in this field. https://supermanherbs.com/ep28-micronutrients/

In my opinion, from talking to them and extensively looking at what is available on the market, Nutrience is the best available multivitamin and mineral supplement of this nature. http://legendarystrength.com/go/multivitamin

This gives a good dose of all the micronutrients, the absolutely critical ones and the lesser ones for testosterone, in their best forms as is known today. Basically it will ensure you have all these bases covered.

Here's the truth. Just one deficiency of something critical like zinc, could stop all your other efforts from working.

Step 3 - Sunshine and Vitamin D

Unfortunately, D got named a vitamin, and thus we tend to think of it this way. But really it should not be, because vitamin D is not really a vitamin at all. It's actually a hormone, or a hormone precursor. It's also unusual, from other vitamins, in that the main way to attain it is from the sun, rather than diet. It is known as the "sunshine vitamin" as we synthesize it in our bodies from sunlight on the skin. Like plants we do our own form of photosynthesis.

The problem is very few people get sunlight anymore for two reasons. One we've been taught that sunlight is bad and causes cancer. Secondly, our civilization has moved just about everything indoors.

Sunlight ought to be thought of as necessary for health. Would you go without food? Would you go without water? Would you go without breathing? But do you go without sunlight?

When getting sunlight, the body synthesizes D from cholesterol and sulfur creating vitamin D3 sulfate. This form is different than what you find in most supplements. (It also indicates the need for cholesterol and sulfur in your diet. This could be why some people don't adequately produce vitamin D despite getting sun.) The unsulfated form in your body requires LDL, the so called bad cholesterol, to transport. But the sulfated form can travel freely throughout the blood stream. The body cannot convert vitamin D3 into vitamin D3 sulfate.

Sulfur can be found in high quality, complete proteins, as it is involved with the amino acids, methionine and cysteine. Good sources of sulfur include most beef, fish, poultry, eggs, as well as garlic, onions and some of the cruciferous vegetables like kale and Brussels sprouts. It can be supplemented with MSM. (You'll notice most of these are repeats from what has already been recommended for other reasons.)

It doesn't take long to generate your own vitamin D, only half the time it generally takes your skin to turn pink. Of course, this does depend on the darkness of your skin, the intensity of the sun and what part of the earth you're on.

But this process can be stopped. First of all, most sunscreens block this from happening (in addition to having xeno-estrogenic chemicals in them). Secondly, this form of D is water soluble and stays on the surface of the skin for about 36-48 hours. If you use soaps on your body during this time you can wash off any of the D you've created.

While you can supplement with D, it's important to note that this isn't the only thing you get from sunlight. Another molecule created is cholesterol sulfate. You also produce nitric oxide. More and more research is coming out on the other benefits of sunlight beyond D, and likely will continue to be revealed in the future.

By all means supplement with D as it is critical for health, including hormones, but the best bet is to transform your lifestyle into a way you can get some daily sun.

That being said, dietary vitamin D is important too. Weston A. Price when looking at the diets of all indigenous peoples, found that vitamin D occurred in all different diets. From the Inuit, where there was almost no sun, to African tribesman that had sun daily, dietary vitamin D was still attained. And none of these people lived all day indoors like we do. Another non-animal dietary option is some mushrooms, like shiitake, when left out in the sun, which also create vitamin D.

Unless you pay lots of attention to getting adequate sun, or eat liver, fatty fish and lots of egg yolks, regularly (which are all decent sources of D), you probably won't have ideal levels so this is one thing worth supplementing with. The Vitamin D Council recommends 1000 IU's per 25 pounds of bodyweight.

You can get your blood tested for 25-hydroxy vitamin D (aka 25-OH-D). Avoid the inaccurate 1.25-dihydroxy test. The normal range is about 20 nanograms/milliliter to 50 ng/mL, while optimal is generally considered to be 50-80ng/mL. This test can be ordered by anyone, not just doctors, from DirectLabs.com.

So now let's look deeper at why vitamin D is important for hormone health, specifically.

One study looked at the correlations of sufficient, insufficient and deficient vitamin D levels in men and how this correlated with androgens. This showed a statistically significant association between the two.

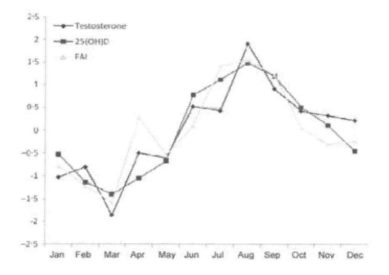

First of all, as you look at the chart above, when does vitamin D naturally go up? In the summer months, with the seasonally longer days, and when people spend more time outdoors.

Another mechanism of action may be that more light lowers melatonin, triggering the pituitary to produce more LH and FSH, in these seasons. This would provide for an association between the two. However, in deficient men, as looked at in another study, more D lead to direct increases.

Another study looked at the direct effect of vitamin D supplementation on testosterone levels. Participants were given 3332 IU's of D3 daily for a year or a placebo. In the supplemental group there were significant raises in both the vitamin D levels in blood and in testosterone (both total and free forms).

It's not known all the exact ways in which vitamin D interacts with testosterone. Seeing that vitamin D works on so many different things it not surprising. But its interaction with cholesterol, which is the starter molecule for all androgens, is one of the possibilities.

Get sun if you can. If not, and possibly even so, this is one thing most people should be supplementing with.

Step 4 – Cell Receptor Health

Imagine this. You have all the testosterone you may need, freely floating throughout your body. Your hormone tests are coming back fine. But you're still suffering symptoms of low T. What is happening?

It's not just about the hormones. But these hormones must be able to signal, or talk to, your cells. Different cells have receptor sites for things like hormones and neurotransmitters. If a cell is supposed to receive testosterone, but the receptor is unhealthy, or blocked, then that testosterone can't do anything.

The above case isn't likely. If the cells are not working properly or are blocked, then chances are this would lead to bad numbers at least over time. But this is another very important different angle to look at.

First of all note that cell membranes are made of fat. A membrane is not just a bag meant to hold everything inside, and keep things out. Instead the cell membrane is the method of communication for cells. Various things come and go inside and outside of the membrane, while others just "talk" to receptors on the outside.

In either case the health of the cell membrane is critical. What is the membrane largely made of? Fat. Saturated fats. Omega 3 long-chain fatty acids, most specifically DHA. And choline as was previously mentioned.

The quality of the fat you're getting is what your cells are made up of.

Instead if we look at the fat sources of most people what do we see. Partially hydrogenated vegetable oils. The partial hydrogenation process is a scary one. Basically if something was fully hydrogenated it almost takes on a plastic-like structure. And that means consuming these things makes your cells built out of the same. It's no wonder we have various forms of resistance on the cell level.

Cells need both the structure of good quality saturated fats, solid at body temperature, and the oiliness of oils like olive oil and fish oil.

Here's the good news and the bad news. If you've been living off of partially hydrogenated oils as well as other rancid, deodorized, omega 6 heavy vegetable oils, you can make a change. Some people have literally called this an "oil change" for the body.

The bad news is that replacing every cell in your body takes time. Some estimate it takes about two years to do so. Of course some cells replace quicker than others. And this will depend on your diet.

All the more reason to get a good amount of fat, of the highest quality possible, on a daily basis.

That covers one part of the equation. The other part is that these cell receptor sites can be blocked by things other than what you want in them.

The various estrogenic chemicals we've discussed will do this. Supporting your elimination of these anti-androgens, and the detox of them is critical.

And there is this other more advanced method using iodine.

This involves the direct application of iodine to the scrotum. The idea is that application, which will absorb through the skin, will provide direct detoxification of the halides (chlorine, bromine, fluorine) as well as radioactive iodine that can block or impair cell receptors. This use of iodine will then support androgen activity. Instead of, or in addition to, taking oral iodine why not apply it to where you want it to go?

After hearing about this protocol I then stumbled upon the following ad in a fitness magazine of the 1930's. Apparently this is not a new idea.

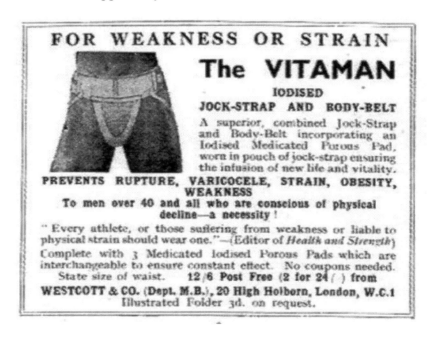

I couldn't find anyone making these jockstraps anymore, but I did come across a specific protocol of supplements to take in addition to painting the iodine on your balls. The reason for these are to help remove the halogens from your body, i.e. supporting their detox. If you push them out with iodine but don't have the other components they can just be reabsorbed.

Although supplements are recommended I think with careful dietary measures you can be sure to have adequate supplies of what is needed. If you do this after a well-rounded multi-vitamin and mineral supplement you should be fine. That is except for the niacin is a larger amount that can't really be gotten from diet alone, which is useful for driving circulation and can be used in detox protocols.

- 100mg Vitamin B2
- 500mg Vitamin B3 or Niacin
- 2000mg Vitamin C
- 200mcg Vitamin K2
- 200mcg Selenium
- 400mg Magnesium
- ½ tsp Sea Salt

After taking these, apply 4-8 drops of an iodine solution to your scrotum and massage it in. Also take 2-4 drops orally at the same time. Allow it to dry sufficiently before putting clothes on. Doing this after a hot shower is useful for opening up the pores. Warning: this can burn!

In addition to the above protocol, I've experimented with just applying a little iodine, like two drops, onto the balls every other day regularly. This does appear to be bringing about a positive effect. This goes along with some of the other ideas in the later section on your relationship with you balls.

In addition to supporting the health of the androgen receptors, what we do may also influence the quantity of receptors in the cells. This does occur with other endogenous chemicals and their receptor sites so it is likely here too. As for what specifically may lead to this I am not sure, but chances are that supporting your health in all the other ways covered here could do this too.

Step 5 - Increase LH and Other T Precursors

As we established near the beginning of this book, luteinizing hormone is what travels from the pituitary to the testicles and begins the cascade of androgen production resulting in testosterone. Thus this can become a focus when we want to boost T.

Most of the herbs that are said to increase testosterone seem to work largely by this pathway (or by fighting the anti-androgens as discussed previously).

There seem to be a variety of foods and herbs that help to do this. In one study, ginger increases LH by 43.2% and increased T by 17.7% in infertile men.

Spinach is full of phytoecdysteroids. Ecdysteroids are hormones that are found in insects and plants, which the human body can use in different ways. The science is still just beginning to investigate this. While there may not be a direct hormonal action, an uptake of protein synthesis does occur. It appears that Popeye knew what he was talking about! Quinoa is another good source of ecdysteroids.

So you see there are quite a few foods that can be helpful. I've seen lists of 101 T-boosting foods, or something similar along those lines. Anything can boost T if you're deficient in some of the vitamins or mineral co-factors that are necessary. And there's a ton we don't know about how all the various phyto-chemicals work in our bodies.

One thing you'll notice is that these things are all real foods. You know what doesn't boost T? Candy bars, potato chips and all the similarly processed crap out there.

Real food is going to give you the best base. Then a few targeted things can do much more for you from that foundation. On this note there's one "miracle root" that you ought to know about, tongkat ali, also known as longjack.

In English this translates "Ali's Walking Stick". And they weren't talking about an actual stick from a tree! It reminds me of that scene from Austin Powers 3 where Mini Me is described as a tripod. It is the root of a tree that grows in Indonesia and Malaysia, where it is highly revered.

Tongkat Ali has been shown to restore testosterone levels, as well as lower estrogen and SHBG. It boosts several parameters of sexual performance, including erectile function, hardness, performance, and satisfaction, and so much more.

In addition to increasing luteinizing hormone, it's also been said to stop the negative feedback loop that would normally shut down this increased production.

What's highly significant is that Tongkat Ali appears to work through three of the mechanisms needed to ensure hormonal health in men:

1. Restore testosterone levels through LH
2. Anti-estrogenic by lowering aromatase
3. Lowers SHBG

Just about every guy that gets on Tongkat Ali is wowed by it because it's such powerful stuff. This has quickly become by second favorite T boosting herb that I've used. Find out more and find high quality at https://supermanherbs.com/tongkat-ali/

(Warning: because this root works so well it has become heavily marketed and there is lots of inferior forms that do not work as prescribed available.)

My favorite is covered in the next page as it can directly supply testosterone and other androgens.

Step 6 - Increase Testosterone Directly

Most of the methods of testosterone increase, at least when it comes to diet, work through alternative methods instead of working on testosterone directly.

But there is one exception to this. Pine pollen is the only somewhat readily available herb that directly supplies androgens. There are probably a lot more out there, it's just that no one has been researching this subject until very recently. Most people interested in health have heard of phyto-estrogens, but very few people know about phyto-androgens.

Pine pollen has a number of androgenic compounds inside, in addition to its wide range of vitamins, minerals and antioxidants.

Some of these compounds are brassinosteroids, which have been shown to be powerful growth stimulators in plants. At least two of these have been shown to help remove estrogens and other toxins from the body. This is further helped by other compounds known as glutathione transferases. These also happen to be involved in the synthesis of progesterone and testosterone.

There are also gibberellins which are structurally similar to testosterone. They've been found to bind to androgen receptors and increase androgen production in the body.

But that's not all. Pine pollen actually has the same forms of human androgens. A species of black pine pollen was measured to have in 10 grams, 0.7-0.8 mcg of androstenedione, 0.7mcg testosterone, 0.1 mcg DHEA, and 0.2 mcg androsterone. These are small amounts but remember that it doesn't take much.

About seven mg of testosterone is produced a day in the average male. So this isn't like getting a shot of testosterone. But with these small amounts, and all the other nutrition pine pollen provides, you can get powerful hormonal effects. That's why pine pollen is probably the first place I'd go for testosterone improvement, with tongkat being a close second. Find more at https://supermanherbs.com/pine-pollen/

One question that I often get about pine pollen, tongkat ali and other hormonal supplement herbs is if it's going to shut down your own testosterone function.

First of all, unless you're doing stupidly excessive amounts, these herbs are nothing like the amounts of hormones in steroids or testosterone injections.

Secondly, these are natural substances, not isolated things. There are all kind of co-factors, vitamins, minerals and other things, which seem to work synergistically with the body to support your own hormones rather than just replace them.

With the stronger hormonal herbs like these two it is still recommended that you cycle them, which is take them for a while then stop doing so. Different people like to do this in different ways. For some five days on and two days off works. For others they'll use the herbs every single day for a month then take a week off. Some do it far more randomly going by how they feel for when they need to take it. Mark Wilson recommends cycling seven different herbs over seven different days. For more information check out this podcast: https://supermanherbs.com/ep14-testosterone-with-mark-wilson/

As always experiment and find what works for you. In any cases, this cycling makes sure to reset the feedback loops in your body. It's not so much for fear of doing any permanent damage, but instead that after you lay off for a while, when you come back on the effectiveness will increase.

That covers supplements for now. So while testosterone is hard to directly influence by diet alone, it's easily changed by what you do in your daily life. Recall the study showing how "power poses," how you sit and stand led to increases in testosterone, while weak postures led to decreases.

Testosterone is about being a man. That means taking responsibility for yourself and for your life. If you do this, then your testosterone will likely increase.

Other manly things do the same thing. Competition is a big one. Watching sports raises testosterone. A study looked at this effect. The interesting thing was that while watching sports, everyone's T increased but the outcome was important too. Fans of the winning team increased in T more, while it dropped for those that lost.

Testosterone production is stimulated by arousal and feeling successful. In contrast, it is known to dip when we get bored, angry, stressed and feel out of control.

While we know you need some testosterone in order to have desire and perform in sexual activity, the opposite is also true. Having sex appears to increase testosterone.

Even watching porn has been shown to increase testosterone by an average of 35% peaking 60-90 minutes after watching. So any erotic stimulation seems to do the trick. However, excessive porn, especially via the internet, has also been linked to dopamine resistance, resulting in something call porn-induced ED. For more info see the later section about the same.

Step 7 - DHT

Recall that DHT is the most potent androgen in our body, far more than testosterone itself. Also important is that it can't be aromatized, and may even inhibit aromatization by itself too. While DHT, like anything, can be in excess, optimizing your DHT will give you the androgenic affects you desire.

Although aromatase can't affect it, DHT can still be bound by SHBG. With that note, realize that anything that lowers SHBG will likely assist in optimizing the DHT you do have.

According to Dr. Carruthers, DHT is not the primary hormone for libido, instead having some of the other effects, which T often gets its reputation from. Recall that DHT is somewhere are 10-50 times as androgenic as T, depending on who you ask. Thus if you want the benefits of testosterone, it may actually be DHT that you want.

Testosterone is converted into DHT via the enzyme 5-alpha reductase, of which there are three different types which appear to have slightly different types and sites of activity. There are number of foods and herbs that increase or decrease this enzyme.

Most of the information out there about DHT has to do with its connection to male pattern baldness, or androgenetic alopecia, of which there does appear to be a DHT link. Yet it's not so simple that if you have too much DHT you will be bald. If that were the case then growing teenage boys would be the ones going bald, when these hormones are typically at their peak.

Research shows that most men with male pattern baldness have low total testosterone, but with more of it free and more of this enzyme and thus DHT. It is also suggested that higher prolactin levels as well as metabolic syndrome or insulin resistance play a role.

In an attempt to fight this, many men have taken the drug, finasteride. Unfortunately this drug has now been linked to long term adverse effects including sexual function. They even have called it post-finasteride syndrome.

The other issue of DHT has to do with prostate cancer and BPH (benign prostate hyperplasia). Here we see difficulties with urinating because as the prostate grows in size it can put pressure on the urethra. This can mean:

- Dribbling (lack of pressure)
- Painful urination
- Frequent urination
- Difficulty starting urination
- Decreased force or urination
- Bladder fullness despite urination
- Nocturia (need to urinate at night)

- Incontinence

Along with these issues, there can be a higher incidence of bladder infections as the urine stagnates.

The prostate is normally the size of a chestnut or walnut but can become as big as a grapefruit (stage IV BPH). BPH appears to be independent of cancer, meaning that it doesn't turn cancerous at some point.

On the other hand, prostate cancer brings about similar symptoms as BPH early on. Later, worse symptoms like blood in the urine, weight loss, bone pain and fatigue can occur.

As in any cancer, in time, it can spread to the rest of the body, ultimately causing death. However it does seem to be a particularly slow growing cancer at least in most cases. Over 30 percent of men that die over the age of 80 and are autopsied are found to have prostate cancer. Because of its slow-growing nature, when it is detected, it is often just watched instead of treated via surgery or radiation.

PSA, or prostate-specific antigen, is a glycoprotein found in the blood that is used for screening prostate issues. Increased PSA levels indicate cancer in about 70 percent of cases. Healthy readings are close to zero, while BPH can be around 4 ng/dL. Levels above 10, or especially 20, show increased cancer risk. The range between 4 and 10 is a bit of a gray zone. Here they often measure free PSA. The higher the ratio of free:total PSA the better off you are.

However, it is important to note that this is not full-proof. There are both false positives and false negatives associated with this test. The other form of testing that is typically used is a rectal exam. As the prostate can be felt a short way up the rectum its size, or growths on it, can be manually felt for. The size of the prostate can also be measured via a transrectal ultrasound.

For a long time DHT, was blamed for BPH. This is because when testosterone enters the prostate, 95% of it is converted into DHT and then binds to the receptor sites there. And it is DHT that causes growth after birth and during puberty.

However, since that time it has largely been vindicated, though this is not common knowledge. If high DHT was the problem, 20-year-olds would have BPH not 50+ year olds.

One longitudinal study found no correlation between testosterone levels and either BPH or prostate cancer. And another study found a high normal testosterone level is one of the best indicators of prostate health. The fact is most studies looking at men with BPH or prostate cancer have normal, or even low, levels of DHT.

So why the confusion? DHT does stimulate the growth of the prostate but most of the time this is kept in check. It appears to be more of a correlated factor rather than a causative one, thus trying to treat prostate issues by lowering DHT is barking up the wrong tree.

What appears to be more at the cause is a higher amounts of estrogen. This is both endogenous as well as exogenous estrogen, and likely other forms of endocrine disruption. A Japanese study clearly found associations of estrogen and enlarged prostates. They stated, "An estrogen-dominant environment plays an important role in the development of BPH."

Other studies have found similar results. "Estrogens and estrogen receptor are clearly linked to the development and progression of prostate cancer."

This begins to make more sense. The prostate doesn't just have a high affinity for DHT, it also concentrates estrogens. To understand why it's useful to look at fetal development. In the center of the prostatic urethra is an indentation called the utricle. This is the undeveloped form of the uterus found in men, which retains estrogen receptors. Many of the cells surrounding this issue also have estrogen receptors. Thus doing all the previous steps is likely to help prevent these issues, as well as support health if you currently have them.

Prostate cancer is typically treated with androgen deprivation therapy, also called androgen ablation. Often the androgens are lowered to castration levels. While this is effective in some cases it does not work in others, the cancers becoming androgen independent. More recently treatment also is anti-estrogenic too instead of strictly anti-androgenic.

In Europe, natural treatment of prostate issues is typically done first, before surgical or pharmaceutical means. And in many cases it is more successful. Part of the reason for this is because there is so much confusion surrounding the topic, while nature has wisdom we've only begun to explore.

The first area to look at is deficiencies. If your body doesn't have the right amounts of crucial things your chances of disease, prostate and otherwise, go up significantly.

Various studies have found higher levels of vitamin D reduce just about all cancer risk. Also previously mentioned omega 3 fatty acids, specifically higher levels of blood EPA directly correlating with lower cancer risk.

Zinc is an important trace mineral when it comes to the prostate, in fact more of it concentrates there than anywhere else in the body. Like the thyroid not having sufficient iodine, causing growth of the gland, in this case called goiter, the prostate not having sufficient zinc is likely a causative factor in BPH, causing the growth of that gland. Supplementing with zinc has shown a reduction in prostate cancer.

As before you'll also want to support your liver health as that is crucial for detoxing excess hormones from the body, as well as much else.

And unless you're suffering from prostate cancer there are two commonly recommended male herbs that you might actually want to avoid.

There are several herbs that are known as 5-alpha reductase inhibitors.

Saw palmetto (*Serenoa repens*) is the #1 go-to herb when it comes to BPH. Various studies have shown saw palmetto to be effective in almost 90% of men with BPH, though of course nothing is full-proof.

While saw palmetto's mechanism of action in which it does this is thought to be 5-alpha reductase inhibition, this is looking at it in a very limited way. I think that finding a molecule in saw palmetto that did this led to strengthening the belief that DHT was causative in prostate issues.

But an herb is not its so-called active constituent. There is undoubtedly a whole lot else saw palmetto is doing. Another function is to block binding of DHT, testosterone and estrogens to receptors in the prostate. It is also anti-inflammatory. Classically, it was used for much more than prostate issues. This included with women, including those with PCOS, and as a general endocrine system tonic affecting the adrenals and the nerves, plus even more.

It is best used as a high percentage alcohol tincture as the active part appears to be better transferred this way than in water, and it doesn't taste good. Very acrid. Best effects are with several months of use, or even longer.

Nettle root (*Urtica dioica*) is also widely used when it comes to BPH. It does appear to have some 5ar inhibiting activity, but we also note that it lowers sex hormone binding globulin and aromatase enzyme. These in turn mean that you have freer testosterone and less estrogen.

More specifically with the prostate, nettle root has been shown to improve urine flow, reduce frequency, and allow for more complete evacuation.

A combo of nettle root and saw palmetto, in a double-blind placebo-controlled study, found a reduction in symptoms and size of the prostate. It performed as well as the drug finasteride, but with far fewer side effects.

I'd also like to mention pine pollen. While there are no studies on it yet for working on prostate issues, I've heard lots of anecdotal evidence. Its mechanisms for action are yet to be known.

Fenugreek is another herb that limits 5-alpha reductase. While it has been shown to increase testosterone, it looks like the mechanism by which it achieved this was by limiting conversion to DHT.

Some other herbs and nutrients which also have 5-alpha reductase inhibitor activity include safflower, astaxanthin, catechins in green tea, rice, and, I was sad to see, reishi mushroom, through the ganoderic acids, which come out more in an alcohol extract rather than a water extract.

Is this all bad though? It appears that even zinc reduces this enzyme. Chances are that several of these things modulate it more, than they directly reduce it. Hopefully, we'll see more information on this topic, besides just for baldness and prostate health, in the future.

Another herb, used for thousands of years in Chinese medicine, is cistanche. Besides having a phallic shape which indicates what it can be used for, this has been shown to lead to increases in both T and DHT, at least in one rat study, where supplemental cistanche doubled testosterone. Find more at https://supermanherbs.com/cistanche/

A few other possible DHT helpers include creatine, sorghum and boron. Probably the most important part of increasing DHT is working out. Although I've called it *T-Boosting Workouts*, the application on DHT may be the even more crucial part.

While there is limited information on what specifically helps to optimize DHT, remember to look at the bigger picture. Although we've focused on one component of hormone health at a time, everything we've talked about here is working in multiple levels.

Establish a Healthy Relationship
with Your Cock and Balls

Now that we've discussed lots of options, foods, herbs and supplements, for battling anti-androgens and stimulating your androgen allies, it's time to focus on your biggest and best ally. Your cock and balls!

Let's start with the balls. Recall that the testicles produce 95% of the testosterone in the male body. One of the health ideas that I've begun to explore further is that to think of ourselves as just a single body is not the most helpful idea.

For instance, more and more is coming out every day about how your gut flora impacts just about every factor of health, most likely even your testosterone production too. Some rodent research has stated the "microbial community alters sex hormone levels" and "the gut microbiome can modulate the permeability of the blood testis barrier and might play a role in the regulation of endocrine functions of the testis."

Surely some bacteria produce chemicals that raise or inhibit testosterone and estrogen, if not creating these hormones themselves. This means good testosterone production requires fermented foods. Real sauerkraut not only can provide beneficial bacteria, the prebiotic fiber for your own, but also many of the benefits of cruciferous vegetables too.

The bacteria cells that reside inside your body, not to mention every other place on your body like your skin too, outnumber your human cells 10 to 1. We're actually more them then we are us.

Furthermore, the human cell has multiple parts. One of these, the power generator of your cells is the mitochondria, which is in every cell. It is believed that long ago, at some point in evolution, the mitochondria were a bacteria which joined with others in order to produce cells like we now have.

Then these cells get together, in order to work together for a higher level function. Each organ you have, the testicles included, is one of these groupings. And the sum of the parts is greater than the parts, but that doesn't mean we should forget about the parts.

I say all this to instill in you the idea that **if you want great testosterone production you need to have a healthy relationship with your balls**.

And on that note some of the things suggested here may be outside the box, just hopefully not too outside the box.

Cold Temperatures

One of the topics discussed earlier was how the testicles descend outside of the body so they can exist at a colder temperature.

So it's important to support this goal. Wear loose fitting cotton or silk boxers. Or probably even better, though possibly with some social stigma, would be to go "free-balling". Several studies have shown decreased sperm production and motility with tight underwear. There's a good chance that testosterone production goes down too. Recall that FSH, comes down from the pituitary, along with LH, to focus more on that sperm producing aspect. If that gets impaired chances are the other pathway might too.

And on the note of colder temperatures, if you want to stimulate this production (of both sperm and testosterone) even more, then use the directly application of cold to the balls. While several people have focused on how application of ice and cold can help your body to burn fat through the activation of brown fat tissue (which helps optimize testosterone itself), it's also been shown that cold or ice on the balls can increase testosterone.

Of course, you don't want to do so much that it causes damage. Be reasonable with it. But if you can withstand the shocking cold on your balls you're manlier and thus will become manlier.

Sunlight

Another useful direct application on the balls is sunlight. Yes, I'm telling you to go tan your nuts!

As beneficial as sunlight is to the body, think about when the last time you ever got sunshine in the places where the sun doesn't shine. If you're like most people it probably wasn't since you were a tiny child and your parents let you walk around naked outside.

As was found by Abraham Myerson, direct sunlight on the scrotum, including the rest of the body, led to significant testosterone increases.

Part of this may be psychological. Remember how we talked about the metaphorical nature of hormones. If you can lay there to tan your balls, you're in a safe and comfortable place and feeling manly, to be completely free.

And as we saw, vitamin D has a connection to testosterone. Getting vitamin D production directly in that area appears to be even more powerful. It's a hormone pre-cursor after all. This just takes it one step further.

Of course, for many people this may not be feasible, but if you could find a way, even to do it once in a while, how would you?

Be prepared for something weird to occur when you try this. I have no clue why this happens, though I take it to mean something positive, but the balls move of their own accord when exposed to sunlight. It startled me when I first experienced it. Then I heard other people talk of the same thing. It must be that the balls like the sun exposure!

Topical Applications

The skin on the scrotum is thin, allowing testosterone, and likely much else to pass through. In fact, the scrotal skin is rich in the enzyme 5-alpha reductase which converts testosterone into DHT while it is being absorbed.

We already talked about direct application of iodine to the balls. What else could possibly be put on them to assist in hormone production? I've done a little work with putting pine pollen tincture there, rather than in my mouth. Anecdotal evidence so far seems to be positive.

Olive oil and coconut oil help the testes absorb more cholesterol to begin their hormone production. This was shown in a study feeding the oil to mice. But if eating these fats directly helps the Leydig cells to use cholesterol, as well as boost the antioxidant concentrations in there, would topical application help? I offer these not as proven techniques but to get you thinking about some new ways you might support your balls.

Cell Phones

One thing worth avoiding is keeping your cell phone in your pocket. Several studies have shown that this leads to lower sperm counts. Chances are it also is going to affect hormone production too.

Limit your use of a cell phone overall. And if you must carry a phone with you, turn it off or put in on airplane mode if it needs to go into your pocket. Or at least carry it in a different pocket, not next to your most sensitive area.

Holding Them

It appears that the testicles do not have strong powers of regeneration, like the liver does. It is well put in *Testosterone Revolution*, "The liver forgives and forgets, but the testis harbors grudges."

But perhaps this can be improved with a healthy relationship. The fact that the Western world has a very odd love-hate relationship with sex, has most of us never thinking about our balls except when in the act, and that can then be clouded by shame and guilt often. In fact, even in sex it's all about the dick, and most aren't concerned with the balls at all.

I believe that any testosterone optimizing plan, to be the best, should include some form of thinking about and holding your balls. What follows next includes just that.

Energetic HPG Axis Drill

In my studies of energy medicine there are a number of ways to energetically correct and help optimize the hormones. I've seen these drills help quite significantly. However, as the system I got involved with was developed by a woman, and 95% of the people involved were women, there was a bent toward the feminine. Some drills involved holding the points over the ovaries and the womb.

As I was practicing with a person, going through this protocol it occurred to me to simply switch it up to the corresponding part. So instead of holding points over the ovaries that I didn't have, I grasped my balls. Since that time I've played with several variations of this drill coming to what seems to work best. As the testosterone feedback look happens primarily through the hypothalamic-pituitary-gonadal-axis you can cover this whole area with just two hands.

Place your left hand over your testicles. This can be over clothing or with skin to skin contact. The right hand comes to rest on the back of your head, with the fingertips pointing forward, right about at the midline of the skull. In this position you're covering the area of both the hypothalamus and pituitary.

Holding these two areas, breathe deeply, while you feel the connection on this axis. I like to imagine and feel a figure eight pattern moving between the two areas. You may notice yawning as a sign of an energetic hook-up. If you don't, hold for up to three minutes.

You can then switch your hands so that the left hand is on the front of your forehead up reaching up to your crown. And then the right hand grasps your balls. I've included this drill as part of the *T-Boosting Hypnotic Visualization* track I put together.

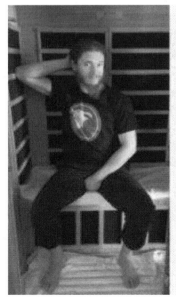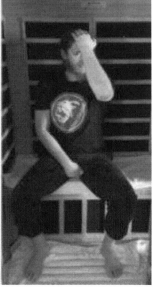

Three Thumps

The above is the main drill, however there are a couple preliminaries that may help it to be more effective. I do these energy drills along with others each day in my morning sauna, as pictured here, except my clothes are usually off.

Rub or thump on your K-27's. These are at the end of the Kidney Meridian (the 27th acupressure point). The kidney meridian, and rubbing these points specifically, will act as a jump start to all the other meridians, thus getting your energies running. This point is right at the end of the collarbone, down about half an inch, and inside about half an inch. There should be a slight indentation there.

When you're doing this, you want to cross your hands because it's natural for the energy of the bodies to crossover. So this just makes sure that you're not throwing off your energies in a different way.

Using two or three fingers massage that area fairly deeply. It may hurt. That's fine and it means that you need to do it.

The next point is on over the thymus gland. Using the five fingers of one hand thump yourself over the middle of the sternum.

The final point has to do with the spleen meridian, known as SP-21. Simply move your hands to the sides of your rib cage a few inches over the bottom rib.

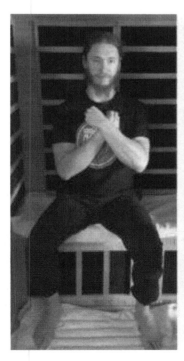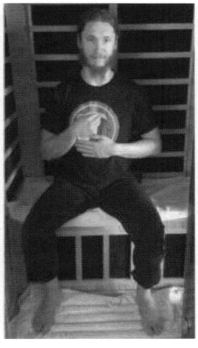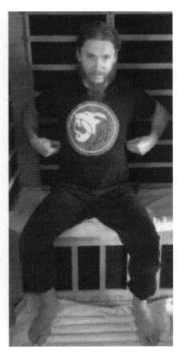

Wayne Cook

The next drill we have here is known as Wayne Cook. It is preferable, but not necessary, to take off your shoes for this. Sit down. Again, we're going back to the kidney meridian except on the opposite end. K1 is located in the middle of the bottom of the foot. It's known as the Bubbling Spring point and it has a whole bunch other names because it's really important point. Bend your leg and rest it across the other knee.

Using the arm on the same side as the leg, take the hand using the middle of the palm and place it over K1. Because your leg is bent you'll be reaching across your body. Take your free hand and rest it on the ankle.

As you do this breathe deeply, look up and smile. If you feel a yawn coming on that is good. It means the energy is hooking up. You'll want to accentuate it. After you feel this hook up or after several breathes switch to the other side.

The final step is bringing the fingers together, the thumbs touching. Place the tips of the thumbs over the third eye area. Take a few breaths in this position.

This drill is great for getting the energies to crossover and to coordinate both sides of your brain.

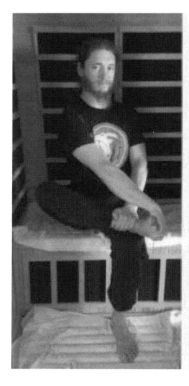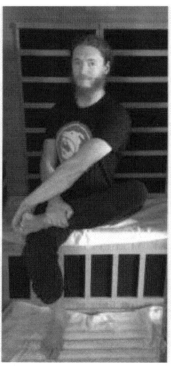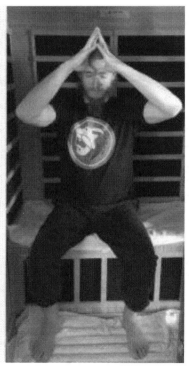

Crown Pull

From the final step of the Wayne Cook it's easy to go into the crown pull. Move your fingers of both hands to the middle of the forehead and pull across towards the sides of your head with pressure against your skin.

After you've done your forehead move them up further on your head and repeat. Keep going until you've done your entire skull and down your neck. After you've finished at the neck place your fingers behind your traps and hold with pressure there. After doing this for a breath or two drag them forward as you breathe out.

This drill helps to energetically, and even physically, make space in your skull. It's very useful to do before the following drills as it sets you up for the following drills, allowing the endocrine organs to communicate better.

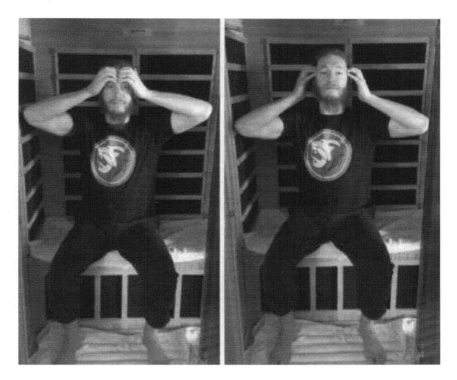

Rooster Crown

The rooster crown is the energetic drill to connect your hypothalamus, pituitary, pineal and the liver. It's called the rooster crown because in some ways it resembles the comb of a cock (and by that I mean the bird).

Both hands are placed on the head. You might be asking how this then involves the liver? Right on the hairline are liver neurovascular points, which connect to the liver meridian.

Place your left hand with the palm on your forehead and the fingers reaching towards the top of your head. Your right hand grasps the back of your skull, with the fingers pointing up the top of your skull again. Depending on how big of a head you have, as well as the size of your hands, they could overlap or not even touch. It's fine in either case.

As you hold this position breathe deeply a few times.

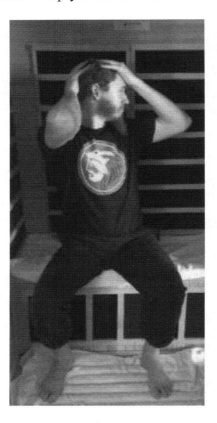

From this point, now move onto the HPG Axis drill, as previously described. That is move your left hand onto your balls and keep the right hand in the same place.

Now Onto Your Cock...

First of all, can you talk about it in such terms? Sure, you only want to do this in the appropriate company, but some men seem so emasculated they can only refer to it as the clinical and politically correct, penis.

As mentioned in Sheri Winston's *Women's Anatomy of Arousal*, we don't have good words to talk about this stuff. It's either considered dirty, too clinical or just plain silly. You'll notice I've used penis, cock, and dick spread throughout this book. It kind of depended on the context, and hopefully I've interjected some humor about it.

But I'm serious about this matter. A real man isn't ashamed about his dick and his desire to use it. Once again, this can be taken to the point of 'assholeness' which we want to avoid. But in the appropriate circumstances you best be able to man up.

You'll notice there's a lot less information here about your dick than the balls. That's because guys do show some love for their dick but tend to neglect the balls. And after all, the balls are what produce the testosterone. The cock is more for using it!

We already talked about the morning wood test and all the helpful insight that can bring. Of course, your performance in sex would be another sign.

(It's not just about testosterone though. Although that's a big piece, there are several other factors that can lead to loss of performance. Lower levels of testosterone are needed to maintain libido than to maintain potency. Dr. Carruthers found in his patients, using TRT, significantly improved in erectile function in 70% of cases. The other 30% did not improve from testosterone alone. In other cases you'll have to look from the psychological, to the dopamine resistance brought about by porn, to the cardiovascular, including nitric oxide and the phosphodiesterase enzyme. There are several components to this whole picture.)

Yes the quantity and quality of your erections is an important clue. You can also take a look at the angle of your erection. In general, the higher up it goes the better everything is work. Staying power is another factor.

In fact, these are a leading indicator of health. So if your testosterone is optimized and it's still not working quite like you'd like, definitely look into these other areas.

For example, epimedium, aka Horny Goat Weed, and its active constituent icariin works on the same enzymatic pathway, phosphodiesterase, as Viagra®, sildenafil citrate, does. Of course, even strong extracts aren't the same strength as the isolated drug is. But nor do they tend to have the same side effects.

Besides the testosterone angle there are a number of other things you can do to enhance erectile function.

Nitric oxide, which is largely responsible for causing and keeping the erection, can be enhanced through a number of methods. Little known is that fact that sunlight on the skin not only produces vitamin D, but also NO as well.

Nitrates can be converted by the bacteria in the body into nitric oxide. This calls for having beneficial gut bacteria as well as eating for foods rich in these. While many processed meats have these added to preserve color, what you really want to do is eat your vegetables. Many green leafy vegetables, and most notably beets, can supply these which then can help with NO levels.

There are also many herbs that can help with NO like cistanche, epimedium, amalaki, garlic, cayenne, ginseng and others. You can also take L-arginine, an amino acid, which is an NO precursor.

If fixing your testosterone doesn't fix any erectile issues, then this is the next area that I would look. In addition to erections, NO is critically important for cardiovascular system health.

Related to NO we also can look at PDE5. This is an enzyme called phosphodiesterase type 5. To keep it simple this enzyme basically breaks down NO which can then cause your erection to go away. This enzyme is the way in which Viagra® and other pharmaceuticals of that nature work, by its inhibition.

What is interesting is that horny goat weed, also known as epimedium, has a compound called icariin that also serves this function. Of course, it isn't as strong as the isolated drug, but it still works on this mechanism, as well as increasing NO as previously mentioned.

If you get erections, but they tend to go away, this is an herb I would experiment with.

There is also the dopamine angle. Dopamine is a neurotransmitter that affects testosterone in many ways. It also plays a balancing role against prolactin.

This biggest problem here is the widespread use of internet porn for masturbation. This causes dopamine resistance. With many young people growing up with this many younger people are experiencing ED. In fact this is such a big issue it has become known as Porn-Induced ED.

I'm not making a judgement on porn or masturbation, just that the combo of these two can prove problematic. Ask yourself if you only ever masturbate with porn? And can you maintain an erection and masturbate without porn? These tests may indicate whether this is an issue for you.

You can read more about this issue, watch videos and learn what to do about it at https://supermanherbs.com/porn-induced-ed/

Lastly, there is the psychological issue. This area is really beyond the scope of this book. As we've talked about the mind effects the body and vice versa so this can be very much an issue.

Anyone that has ever had ED even once, even if for any of the other reasons stated above, is likely to then have the psychological issue on top of it.

Depending on the depths this may best be treated with a psychologist or psychiatrist. There are other methods like EFT or NLP that can also help.

That's just a quick overview of some of the other issues at play if ED is an issue for you. I plan to have more in depth information about this and related issues available in the future.

The Testosterone Action Plan and Checklist

We've covered a ton of information. And there's no way you can do it all so don't even think about that. Instead I want to break down this information into an action plan for you. Remember that this is part of the *Upgrade Your Health* series. The big idea behind that is that, no matter where you are at, you can continually upgrade yourself. The goal here is optimized testosterone, and of course that means optimized estrogen, aromatization, SHBG, DHT and more as well.

Since this issue is bigger than most I've done, instead of a simple list, I've decided to break things up into the different big areas and then give you a checklist for each one that encapsulates just about everything from this book. Of course, more could be added but this definitely will give you enough of a simple and advanced place to start with.

Testing
- ☐ Blood or Saliva Test
- ☐ Morning Wood Test
- ☐ Schwing Test

Nutritional
- ☐ High Quality Water
- ☐ Eat Organic
- ☐ Eat Cholesterol
- ☐ High Quality and Good Quantity of Fat (Animal Fat, Butter, Olive Oil, Coconut, etc.)
- ☐ High Quality and Good Quantity of Carbohydrates
- ☐ Good Ratio of Omega 3 to Omega 6 Fatty Acids
- ☐ Eat Cruciferous Vegetables
- ☐ Eat Other Green Vegetables (Celery, Artichokes, Arugula, Spinach, Radish, etc.)
- ☐ Eat Dark Colored Fruits like Berries and Pomegranates
- ☐ Eat Beets or Beet Juice
- ☐ Use Culinary Herbs like Parsley, Oregano, Basil, Tarragon, Turmeric and more
- ☐ Limit Phyto-Estrogenic Foods
- ☐ Limit Heavy Metal Contaminated Foods
- ☐ Limit Myco-Toxin Contaminated Foods
- ☐ Avoid Heavily Processed Foods

Lifestyle

☐ Get Rid of Excess Fat

☐ Self-Responsible, Confident, Positive Mental Outlook

☐ Quality and Quantity of Sleep

☐ Posture and Physiology

☐ Stress Lowering Activities Daily

☐ Sunlight

☐ Non-Chemical Personal Care Products

☐ Minimize Use of Plastic

Supplemental and Herbal

☐ Vitamin D

☐ Zinc

☐ Iodine

☐ Boron

☐ Fat Soluble Vitamins

☐ Full Micronutrients

☐ Methyl Donors

☐ Pine Pollen

☐ Tongkat Ali

☐ Cistanche

☐ Nettle Root

☐ Mucuna

☐ Ashwagandha

☐ Adaptogens

☐ Green Tea

Workout

- ☐ Heavy Strength Exertion
- ☐ Feel Stronger and More Energized When You Finish Training than When You Begin
- ☐ Getting In Touch with the Feelings of Testosterone
- ☐ Squats
- ☐ Deadlifts
- ☐ Overhead Lifting
- ☐ Odd Objects
- ☐ High Strength Bodyweight Training
- ☐ Sprinting

Relationship with Your Balls

- ☐ HPG Axis Drill
- ☐ Loose Fitting Underwear
- ☐ Avoid Carrying Cell Phone in Pockets
- ☐ Cold Water on the Balls
- ☐ Sunlight on the Balls
- ☐ Topical Iodine Protocol
- ☐ Other Topical Ball Treatments?

Developing Your Own Personal Protocol

We can't deny the placebo effect as a possible powerful stimulator of testosterone either. If you intention is to boost testosterone, assuming you're not working from a place of psychological reversal, this intention alone is likely to help.

Hell, reading this book probably has positively influenced your testosterone in some way!

While it's great to have scientific study giving "proof" about what works and what doesn't, not everything can or will get studied. And just because something was found to work for a group of people doesn't mean it will work for you.

My purpose in this book is to point you in the right direction and give you lots (some might say even too many) things to try. Why is this? Because you'll have to experiment to find what works best for you and your body.

I want you to develop your own protocol. By protocol I mean something that involves more than one step. While everyone wants to take the "magic pill", and some of the herbs can act like that at times, by stacking together multiple things you'll surely get even more benefits. High testosterone must become part of your lifestyle.

The *5-Step Testosterone Jump Start* bonus that came with this, is one such example that takes minimum time yet can have maximum effectiveness.

On the SuperManHerbs.com website was left a couple of comments from a man named Alan. I wish to share this with you not so that you can do the exact same thing, though feel free to try it out, but to see an example of what he calls his Super T-booster protocol.

"Upon waking, take at least 5-6 eye dropperfuls of pine pollen tincture and 1-2 spoonfuls of pine pollen. Commence with a rigorous workout, preferably lower body so the groin area gets lots of movement and fresh oxygen. After workout, eat a high protein, low estrogenic breakfast and another tablespoonful of pine pollen. Take a shower and make sure at least the final 10 mins are in cold water – with the cold water directly on testicles. This method works great for me and others to whom I have recommended it. Your T levels will be maxed out throughout the day.

"I cycle this for about 10 days on and the 10 days off. During the "off days" I take 2400 mg of tongkat ali + 1800 mg of high potency nettle extract and 1800 mg of fenugreek. Most guys will shun away from the ice cold showers and it does take some getting used to, but now my body seems to crave the T-spike I get from it. It is the icing on the cake!"

You can see it's a combination of things, from the different areas we've covered. It's not just nutritional. It's not just supplements. It's not just cold water. It's not just working out.

It's all of the above put together in a specific sequence aimed at getting the desired result.

Stack the things you've learned in this book like this and you too can have optimized testosterone at any age.

And when you do please drop me an email at logan@legendarystrength.com. I would love to hear your results, as well as about the protocols you've developed and what works best for you.

Sample Recipes

This is not meant to be a cookbook. And while I think these recipes taste good, I am far from a world-class chef.

Instead I want to show you how you take the above information regarding diet and put it into action in simple, tasty and effective ways. You do not need to prepare these recipes exactly as is, though feel free to do so if you so choose. It's included here more as an idea generator so you can move these foods into your daily life.

With some of them I don't include the directions on time, heat and that sort of thing because how well you like your steak cooked or vegetables steamed is up to you. Plus these are just templates. One thing can often easily be switched out for another.

If lots of the foods mentioned are new to you just work on adding one thing per week, or grabbing one new item from the grocery store each time you go there. In time you can come to have many of these foods as things that you regularly consume.

At that point, that is when you begin to get the real benefits. A single dose of parsley won't change your aromatase, but if you regularly eat it, along with many other similar compounds, that's when the hormones will shift for the better.

Oysters

Because of the high zinc in oysters (not to mention they're loaded with lots of other good stuff like selenium, omega 3's and more) they make my #1 recommendation as a testosterone food. I believe the ideal way to eat these is raw. Adding some lemon juice, horseradish or hot sauce can enhance the flavor.

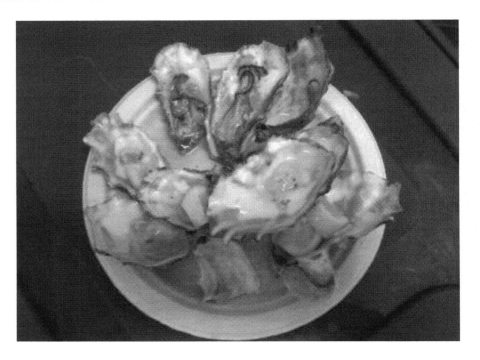

Getting high quality raw oysters isn't always an option. (For that reason about 80% of the time I see them on the menu at a restaurant I'm at I will get some.)

Another option is pre-packaged oysters. You can find these boiled or smoked. I like the ones from Crown Prince since they come in BPA-free tins. They're packed in olive oil and like this one below has chilies added. These are great to have as a snack at home or even take with you when traveling.

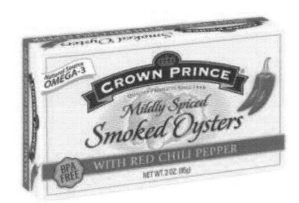

Poached Eggs in Bone Broth and Kale

I haven't mentioned bone broth in this book though it is certainly a powerful health food. Loaded with protein, collagen, vitamins and minerals, it is also a great thing for healing the gut, of which many people do have some healing that could go on there. Vegetable stock would also work. Some from the store may be okay but the best bet is to make your own.

Poach your eggs in bone broth. I picked up this amazing idea from my friend Tyler Bramlett. Everyone that I pass this idea onto, that loves eggs and loves bone broth, thanks me for it.

Get the bone broth boiling in a pot, then break as many eggs into it as you want. Let it continue to boil for 30 seconds then remove from heat. The eggs will continue to cook while it cools. By the time it's ready to eat, the whites should be done, but the yolks still runny.

Add some kale or other greens into the bone broth along with the eggs for a more balanced meal. Feel free to add other vegetables, herbs and spices. Pictured below you'll see kale and some tomato in it as well.

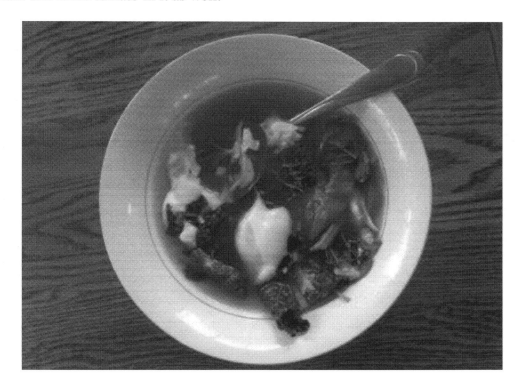

www.LegendaryStrength.com   91

Raw Eggs in OJ with Herbs

This is a great quick meal replacement. I will sometimes use it as a post workout shake as it has a fair amount of carbs and protein, but is made of real foods and doesn't even use protein powder.

You can easily use just the OJ and the eggs, but I often add the following herbs into it. Goji berries and pine pollen are also complete proteins. Pine pollen of course helps with the androgens and goji berries have compounds that help with growth hormone.

- 2 Cups of Fresh Squeezed Orange Juice
- 3 Raw Eggs
- 1 TB Goji Berry Powder
- 1 TB Pine Pollen Powder

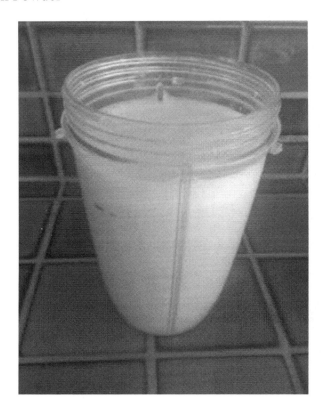

Salmon, Greens and Quinoa

The following shows a complete meal. A good mix of carbohydrate, fat and protein. This is a filet of salmon with a spice rub on it.

Then there is a greens-rich quinoa side. Towards the end of cooking the quinoa in water I added a bunch of veggies from my fridge that needed to be used. In this case it was kale, green onions, parsley and cilantro. I threw in a few pumpkin seeds for extra zinc and doused this preparation in olive oil.

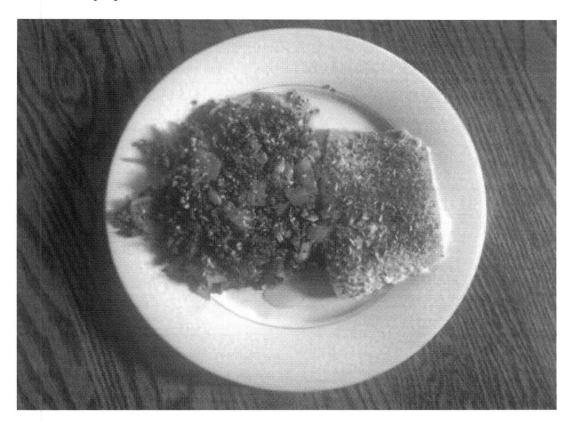

Steak with Buttered Broccoli

This is one of the most basic testosterone supporting meals there is. Simple yet it tastes good and is effective.

Grill a steak, from a high quality grass-fed cow, to perfection. If you want you can use a marinade or spice rub, but often I'll just enjoy this plane.

The side dish is a full head of broccoli with a few tablespoons of butter. I'll often sprinkle some sea salt or the seaweed, dulse, on top of this.

This can be followed with some sort of carbohydrate dish, like some of those mentioned below. Probably my favorite side for this is a sweet potato.

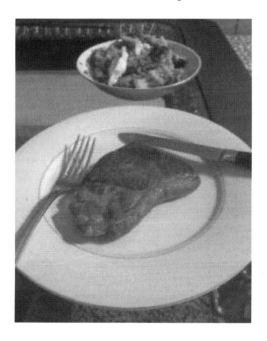

Greens and Butter

Just like the above but another example. Green leafy vegetables become the delivery vehicle for butter. (Just make sure it is butter from grass-fed cows. Fortunately, Kerry Gold is a widely available version of this.)

Here is a bunch of chard, along with the aromatase-fighting parsley, with a fair amount of butter. You can use other fats in place of butter. Sometimes I'll make the same thing but with olive oil or coconut oil.

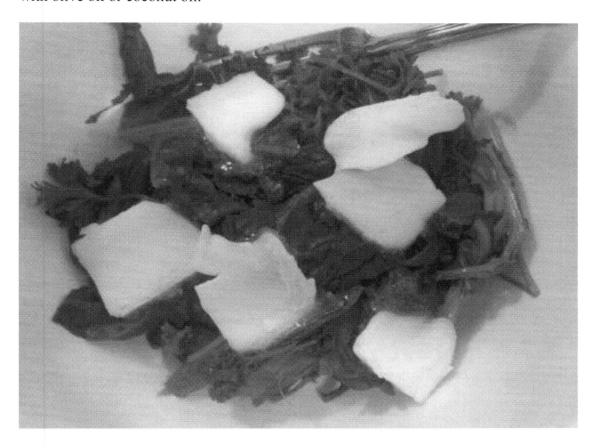

Mashed Cauliflower

What if you could take the cancer-fighting detoxing properties of cauliflower and make something that tastes every bit as good as mashed potatoes? You can!

- One head of Cauliflower
- 1/3rd bunch of Parsley
- 4 cloves of Garlic
- 6 TB of Butter

Steam the cauliflower until it is ready. Then throw it in a blender along with all the other ingredients. A Vitamix, or similar blender, works best as the plunger helps to mix things up. If you don't have one of these you can stop blending, mixed it up with a utensil, blend again and repeat until it is ready. Once it is whipped up it will have a very similar texture as mashed potatoes.

It feels like having a side of carbs, and can be quite filling, but it's a green leafy vegetable. Feel free to do more or less of the above ingredients and to experiment with other ones. Rosemary can taste great in here as well.

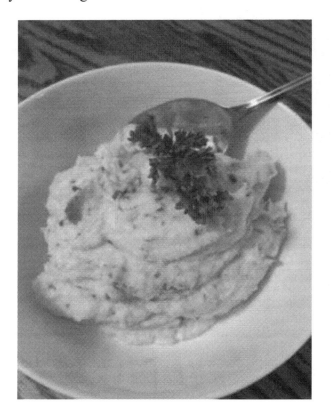

Sweet Potato with Honey and Butter

I often do some version of this with dinner. A standard template for my night time meal is some sort of green leafy vegetables, some sort of meat or fish and then a source of carbs. Sweet potatoes probably tops my list on quality carbs to eat not just for nutrition but taste too.

It can be turned into a dessert dish by adding fat and sugar. Of course here we'll use grass-fed butter and a raw (preferably local) honey. Coconut oil, or coconut butter also makes a good substitution for the butter.

Put the sweet potato in the oven at 375 degrees for about 40 minutes. Once done (which is if you can stick a fork through it easily) put it in a dish, open it up and then add butter and honey. One tablespoon each is a decent amount but you can use more or less.

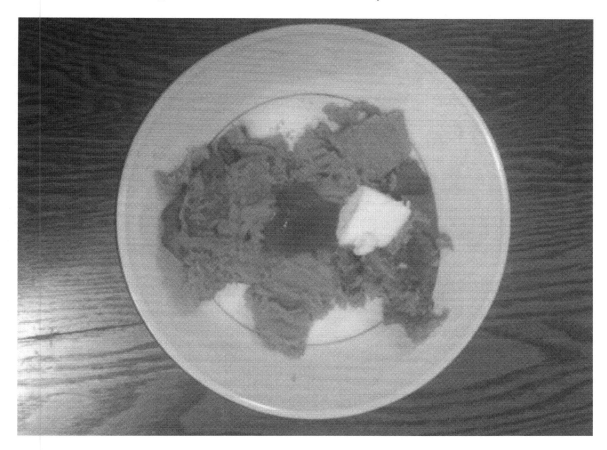

Roasted Beets

For a long time the only way I really consumed beets was in juices. But more recently I've started cooking with them. It's very similar to roasting potatoes, except here you get loads of TMG and other components that assist in your nitric oxide production and detoxification.

Not only that, but beets are sweet. It's not a hit you over the head type of sweetness, but a subtle taste you can enjoy.

They can be roasted in many different ways. Below I cut up a bunch of beets (saving the greens for a different meal later) and put them in a glass dish. I drizzled some olive oil and thyme on them. Then roast them in the over at 375 degrees for about 40 minutes. Once they're ready you can add a little more olive oil and thyme then serve.

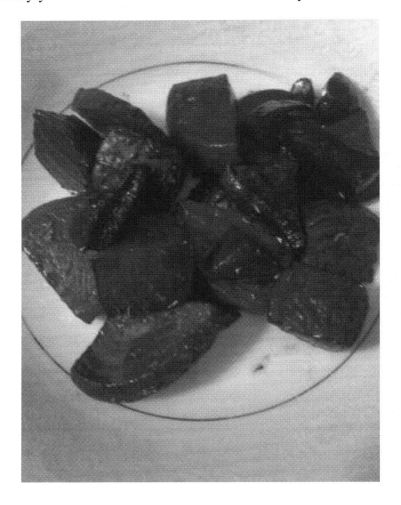

Liver, Bacon and Onions

The benefits of organ meats was only briefly mentioned in this guide. But if you are looking for super foods this is one place you have to look. These are probably the most nutrient dense foods in existence. Also known as offal, you need to learn how to prepare them right so that they taste good.

Liver is fairly easy to get. Of course, you want it coming from healthy animals. With organ meats this is probably even more important than muscle meat.

How do we make liver taste good? Bacon! (Try to get it from pasture raised pigs.) Cooking these together, the liver takes on a bacon like flavor. We'll also add in the often used onions along with it.

Soaking liver in lemon juice or milk can help get rid of the blood which helps in the flavor. Cut up bacon into small pieces and place in a frying pan. Cut up onion and add to the bacon. It is important to not overcook the liver so you'll only want to add this in to the final 3-4 minutes of cooking. If the liver takes on a very chewy texture you've overcooked it.

In the meal pictures below I threw in some fresh turmeric root and white button mushrooms for even more nutritional and hormonal power.

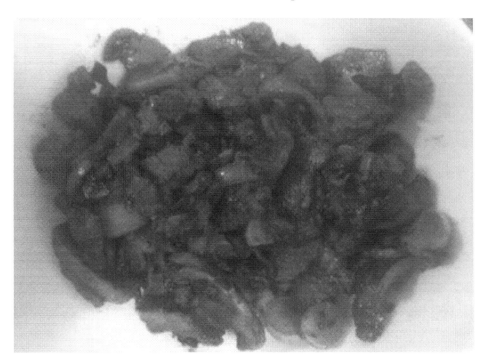

Berry Sorbet

The following is a base recipe that can be turned into a delicious desert. It can be made with a Vitamix blender or with an ice cream maker after blending the ingredients. If you don't have a Vitamix you can sub out the ice for water and then drink it as a smoothie.

- 1 Cup Frozen or Fresh Blueberries
- 1 Banana
- 2 Scoops Whey Protein Powder (from grass-fed cows or goats)
- 1 TB Raw Honey
- 1 cup Ice

This is a great way to add in some herbs for more testosterone support. Here's a few options I've played with but there are many other options too.

- 1 TB Pine Pollen
- 1 tsp Nettle Root
- 1 TB Seabuckthorn Berry Powder
- 1 TB Goji Berry Powder
- ½ tsp Mucuna

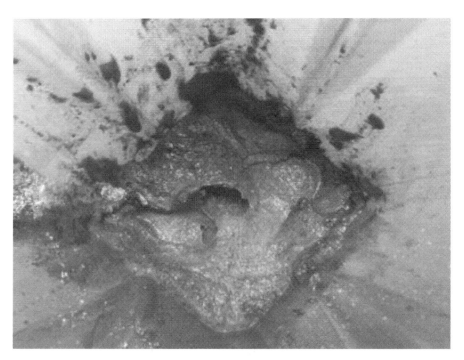

Oats Meal

Oatmeal is interesting. It's thought of as a breakfast grain by many, whereas other ones are often reserved for lunch or dinner. While I try not to eat a whole lot of grains, oats is one that I sometimes make an exception for.

I wouldn't recommend buying instant oatmeal or rolled oats. Instead get steel cut oats or the full oat groats. These should then be soaked in water overnight. This deactivates phytic acid which can impair absorption of certain minerals. After soaking they are actually edible right away, or you can cook them in the soak water. After being soaked they cook much faster too. Instead of 40 minutes or so they can be ready in 10-20 minutes.

Then there are lots of things you can add. Pictured below I had all of the following:

- Handful of Berries
- 1 TB Hemp Seeds
- 1 TB Chia Seeds
- 2 Brazil Nuts
- ½ tsp Mucuna extract powder
- 1 tsp Cordyceps extract powder
- 1 tsp Raw Honey
- 1 TB Coconut Butter
- ¼ tsp Cinnamon

Note that I typically use fresh berries but they were not in season at the time of this picture. Instead I used frozen berries which I added into the oats at the final couple minutes of cooking.

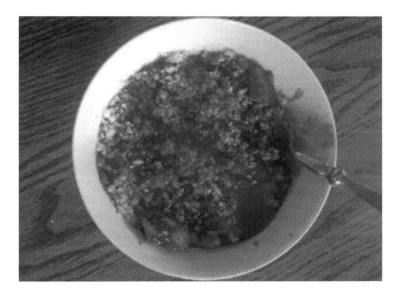

T-Boosting Workouts

While some form of movement is essential for hormonal health, it does seem to be the case that certain exercises and forms of training are best for the testosterone boosting effect. That's what this guide is all about.

While we'll get to specific exercises and workouts, much of the importance for this effect is HOW you do them. Recall from Upgrade Your Testosterone, that the hormones are chemical messengers that work both ways. By having higher T you're going to be stronger and more likely to workout. AND by working out and getting stronger you're going to get higher T.

We'll be exploring some of the research around this at the end. But this section isn't designed to be highly scientific. (I bet that reading research reports could lower T themselves. I wonder if there's any research on that?) Research always lags behind the experience of the people in the field. While I definitely would like to see the ideas in this book all put to the test, it's not likely to happen in a placebo controlled study. In the meantime, your experience and the effects it brings will have to do.

If you grasp some of the principles here than you'll be able to gain this effect just about any time you want. There are three main principles, which we'll go over in detail.

1) Heavy Strength Exertion

2) Feel Stronger and More Energized When You Finish Training Than When You Began

3) Getting in Touch with the Feelings of Testosterone

#1 - Heavy Strength Exertion

This one is pretty self-explanatory. If we're talking about testosterone, for the most part we're talking about heavy weights and big loads. While you can certainly get the effect with other exercises, including the intense bodyweight examples we'll discuss, nothing seems to compare to the nature of a near maximal or maximal load. Here's a short list of the TOP T-boosting exercises in my opinion:

- Deadlifts
- Squats
- Overhead Lifting
- All Kinds of Odd Objects
- Partial Lifts of Any of the Above

In my opinion, some of the very best exercises will be more than maximal by using partial movements. These will all be explained in more depth later on.

What constitutes heavy depends on you and where you're at. You don't have to be lifting record breaking amounts to get T. It's just that it ought to be heavy for you, whatever weight that is. Moderately heavy still works. And as long as you follow the principles of progressive training you'll continue to get better.

Why does this work? Testosterone is the main male hormone. Being strong is a manly thing. Not that women can't, or shouldn't, be strong too, but the fact of the matter is men are stronger by nature. And a woman that works out in this manner is doing something masculine. It's simply the nature of strength. It is a yang activity.

Thus, when you lift something heavy, when you exert your strength, you're boosting testosterone. It's competitive in nature even if you're not in a competition. Its man versus iron (or a rock) and your goal is to win. Simple as that.

Since its heavy, you'll typically be doing smaller rep ranges, usually in the 1-5 range. But you can do more. Partials especially lend themselves to doing higher reps safely. It does appear that as you go over into the strength-endurance zone (like a 20 rep squat or a set of 50 partials) that you go a bit more into growth hormone territory. They still seem to work for T, but you must be more careful not to violate the 2nd principle.

#2 - Feel Stronger and More Energized When You Finish Training Than When You Began

When it comes to training there seems to be two sides. Done one way, training is extremely anabolic. The androgens are anabolic in nature, helping you to build yourself up stronger. This is why testosterone helps build muscle mass as well as stronger bones.

The other side is catabolic, which is a breaking down. Cortisol and its related hormones are of this nature. And training can be heavily catabolic. Marathon runs are a pretty extreme example of this. Here the body is trying to survive, and the long duration runs can have a pretty extreme cost on the body.

But strength training workouts can be much the same way too. Go too long and you'll be wiped out. Do too much volume and you'll be quite sore as the muscular tissue is broken down to be rebuilt later.

These aren't necessarily bad. If you want to build muscle fast then some level of breakdown is needed. And by all means, if you enjoy marathons do them. But don't think they're the best form of training, especially if we're looking at hormones.

CrossFit, is commonly used as a verbal punching bag. While there are some of great things about it, at many boxes, by many people it is often done too frequently, with too much intensity and volume, which can tank testosterone, jack up cortisol, and lead to injuries.

Our goal with training is increasing testosterone in the moment. To do so we don't want to enter catabolism. We do this in a couple of ways.

Keeping the workout to a half hour or 45 minutes max can work. And this is why you see the commonly referenced keep your workouts under an hour advice. For the T-boosting effect I like to go even shorter. Keep the workouts short. This can even be 5, 10, 15 minutes long.

But time isn't the only factor. Some workouts can destroy you in ten minutes. Or that 45 minutes can be lots of rest with only a few minutes of real work. It all depends in how you use the time.

The important part is to feel strong. The *feeling of strength* is one of our primary indicators of testosterone. You may need to warmup and do a few sets to get into the groove. Possibly more important than the actual weight that you lift is whether or not you feel strong when doing it.

Getting to this feeling of being strong is the point of this training. And once you have it you can be done. Sure, you can do a few sets or go for a few more pounds to feel even stronger.

But what we want to avoid at all costs is doing too much where you begin to feel tired or weak. Avoid failure. If you're in a competition with whatever you're lifting you've got to win. Failure is preceded by fatigue. And testosterone is the "success hormone", thus we want everything we do to be successful in the gym.

Contrary to popular opinion you don't need to *force* your body to get stronger or bigger. The body adapts. If you lift progressively, it doesn't matter if you run yourself into the ground (except this comes with a catabolic cost) or if you keep it relatively easy. Your body will adapt either way.

Thus, when you're done training you should feel refreshed. You should feel energized. Much more so than when you began your workout. You should feel like you can do a lot more. These are all signals that testosterone is coursing through your veins.

#3 - Getting in Touch with the Feelings of Testosterone

As we look to the *feelings* of testosterone we have just covered how it relates to feeling strong and energized. But what other feelings go along with this? A few words that describe it might include:

- Animalistic
- Aggressive
- Competitive

- Powerful
- Sexual
- Strong

- Confident
- Energized
- Fun
- Successful
- Manly

And you'll notice some of these have already come up previously. So the idea here is accessing more of these while we train. These, of course, can also be applied outside the gym too.

In being animalistic, you can think of being an animal more than being a man. Look at our distant cousins, the other great apes. These animals are STRONG. Probably have a lot more testosterone too. Or, I've heard several people say, that indigenous men, and our human ancestors from long ago, had two to ten times the testosterone men have today. Try stepping into that *feeling* as you train.

Get aggressive. While I don't think aggression is appropriate for all forms of training, when it comes to testosterone, it is useful. Feel the aggression that could be channeled for war and put it into lifting iron. I've written a whole book on the idea of psyching up, called *Berzerker State: Psyching Up for Strength and Sports*, available at http://legendarystrength.com/berzerker-state/. I highly recommend you check that out for more detail, to learn several ways to amplify your psych-ups. When it comes to partial lifting a good psych-up can literally allow you to lift a hundred pounds more.

Become competitive. While different people seem to be more competitive or less so than others, it does seem to largely be a male trait, with higher T individuals exhibiting more of it. Even if you train alone you can compete against yourself. Or compete against the iron. This is one reason that odd objects are great. They appear to have a life of their own at times, thus it is a bit more of a competition against them.

And if you can include other men and compete against each other, all the better. The important thing is to WIN. While competition brings out testosterone, winning does even more so, with losing causing some loss. So be successful in your competing as much as possible.

Act confident. Know that you will be successful and you will be more so. Real men are confident in what they do (even when they shouldn't necessarily be!) And some research I saw said that over-confident still were more successful than the realistic.

Have fun while doing this. Having optimal testosterone means more enjoyment out of life. So enjoy this process while you're doing it and you'll have more testosterone too. You can do all of the above and below while maintaining a certain playfulness or state of fun while you do so.

Feeling powerful is almost synonymous with strength. Dominant would be another way to describe it. Think back to a time when you were working out and felt as powerful as a god!

Could you be sexual when you lift? No I'm not talking about humping weights. But can you apply that sexual energy into what you're doing. The great success author, Napoleon Hill, described sex as an emotion that can be used for sex, but also for other things like business success if it is transmuted. The same can apply in the gym. Its powerful stuff, so beware using this so much that it drains you.

If you do this all, you will be manly. And that means more T! You don't have to do every single piece of it though. Experiment. Find out what works best for you to access your testosterone and then apply it.

What to Avoid?

It might also be useful to look specifically at what ought to be avoided in training, to give you the flip side of this picture. For some people this may be easier to grasp. Here's a list of things to avoid, when you seek to boost testosterone:

- Failure
- Fatigue
- Exhaustion
- Feeling Weak
- Light Weights
- High Reps
- Lack of Confidence
- Lack of Manliness

I mentioned being energized after your train and avoiding fatigue. Of course, sometimes you'll need to work harder than others. There is a Chinese maxim that says, "It is okay to become fatigued but never exhausted." This is in regards to one of the three treasures, Jing, which is highly correlated along with the sex hormones. It's a good rule of thumb to keep in mind.

Sometimes it is appropriated to work harder and longer than other times and come back from it the conquering hero. This must be modulated and you must find out how often it works for you to go balls to the walls, and when you need to ease back. If you actually compete, that is a time to leave everything on the field, not in every training session.

Exercises

The best exercises for T-boosting training require the use of a barbell, and ideally a power rack. Secondly, a selection of odd objects, which include rocks, barrels, kegs, logs and more, will also work.

This is a personal theory but I believe part of the benefits from testosterone come from not just stimulating the muscles, which is of course very important, but more. The partial exercises also work on the strength of the tendons, ligaments and even bones. These are often neglected areas of training, yet are one of the keys to super strength.

It is well known that weight bearing on the bones makes them stronger. Any sort of weight lifting helps fight osteoporosis for example. This sort of lifting super charges that. Furthermore, I believe that stimulating the bones in this way stimulates your overall vitality in other ways. Partials and supports are the only ways to supra-maximally load the bones like this.

You can make substitutions, using dumbbells and kettlebells, but, they're not the ideal tools for the job, as it's hard to go as heavy with them. That's once you're quite strong. For many beginners these tools will be fine for some of the exercises.

That being said, following the principles outlined above, you can apply those to most forms of training. So what is shown below is just the BEST exercises for the job.

I've also included a few bodyweight options so that there are no excuses. Not everyone has access to a power rack and lots of weights. While not as ideal with the right bodyweight exercise selection as will be outline you can still "go heavy" with these exercises. Thus you can still get many similar effects.

Deadlifts

The deadlift is a great demonstration of your strength. There's just something natural and primal about picking up a heavy weight off of the ground. Hence it works great for our purpose here. It allows you to handle quite heavy loads and works the major muscles in the back and legs. Plus you are able to work this in various forms, variations, and rep and set schemes.

1. Setup a barbell with weight on the ground.
2. Bend down flexing at the knees and the hips. Maintain a shoulder width stance or slightly inside.
3. Grip the bar with a normal grip or reverse grip if going heavy.
4. Maintaining a straight back come to a standing position pulling the bar off the ground.
5. Lower down.

Generally, you do not let your back round. As you get use to the deadlift you may be able to do this, as I personally am, but it should be avoided for safety reasons when you're starting out, and by most people. Also note that I tend to deadlift with a high hip position. Most people will want to start with lower hips than I have in the below picture.

Several other great T-boosting variations include:

* Sumo Deadlift (wide stance with hands inside the legs)
* Jefferson Deadlift (straddling the bar with one foot in front and one behind)

There are lots of other variations, like a one leg deadlift, suitcase deadlift, or a behind the back deadlift, but you tend to use significantly less weight in these.

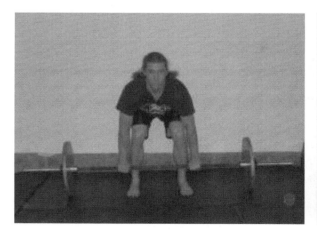 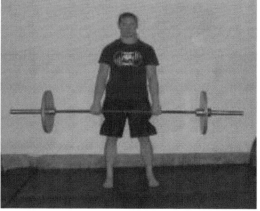

Rack Pulls and Partial Deadlifts

A short range partial deadlift is often also called a rack pull. Some people say that this is always from right above the knees but you can work any range of motion. In my opinion if you're pulling it off the rack, it's a rack pull. For T-boosting, as one of the goals is heavy weight, just a short lockout may be best. As you can see in the picture below I worked up to handling 1025 lbs. in this manner. I can confidently tell you that handling over half a ton, in any manner, makes you feel very manly and strong.

These will work the grip to a big degree so the use of straps is essential as you handle extremely heavy weights. While I don't recommend straps for normal deadlifts, here they are warranted.

1. Setup the barbell in a power rack at the appropriate height.
2. Since you'll be handling heavy weights a reverse grip is a must. The use of straps is highly recommended.
3. Bend the knees slightly and lean forwards at the hips while keeping the arms straight to get into your starting position. Keep the back straight.
4. Pull and stand tall.

Recommended ranges of motion include the top inch or two, a quarter deadlift (above the knee caps), a half deadlift (below the knee caps), and a ¾ deadlift (about mid shin level). Of course, if you have a power rack with more holes, or use some other methods of making the jumps more incremental, you can work all the points in between these.

In working these different ranges of motion you'll find what you're stronger and weaker points in the deadlift are. For me, right around the knees, tends to be the weakest part. Thus, they can be useful in many circumstances for increasing you normal deadlift too, if that is a goal of yours. For others, forget the "full-range" deadlift and you can just do partials as a safer and more effective exercise.

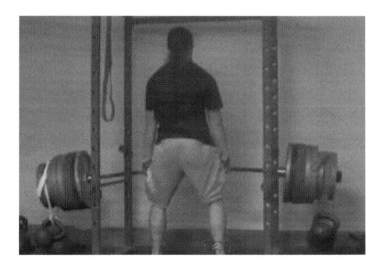

Squats

The squat is known as the king of exercises, for building full body strength and adding on tons of muscle. This is because it targets the legs primarily, the biggest muscles in the body. In addition your body is going to need to support the large weight while the exercise is being done. So for boosting testosterone, it's hard to beat.

1. Using a power rack or squat stands you'll load up the bar with the weight to be used. (Or pick up the barbell from the ground in the Steinborn squat method, another manly exercise.)
2. Get under the bar with it balanced from right to left.
3. Raise it up and step back. It is helpful to breathe in before you descend in order to help stabilize the torso.
4. Get your feet approximately shoulder width apart. Some people like to go a little wider. Find the stance that works for you. You can have parallel feet or shift the toes out a bit.
5. Sit back and down with a straight back, mostly upright. Lower under control.
6. Go until your thighs are parallel or rock bottom in depth.
7. Then stand back up. That constitutes one rep.

Several other great T-boosting variations include:

- Zercher Squat (where you hold the bar in the crooks of your elbows)
- Front Squat (where the barbell is held in front of you)
- Bottom Start Squats (any variation, but you start from the bottom rather than the top)

If you have a limited weight supply or no power rack a substitution can be done with the Bulgarian Split Squat, which focuses on a single leg at a time, but without the balance issues of doing pistol squats.

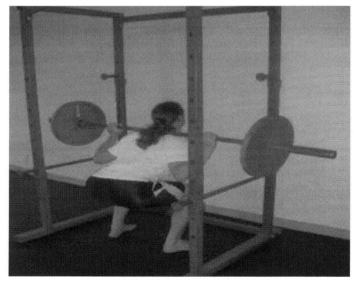

Partial Squats

The partial squat is a powerful hip and thigh developer. Also the back and abs are engaged to a large degree when doing this exercise as you must support the weight on your shoulders. As before with the deadlifts you can do multiple ranges of motion.

In the quarter squat, you will be standing up to lock-out with your knees and your hips from about 5 inches below your starting height. You'll be able to handle a very heavy weight for this once you've become used to the position.

In the half squat and ¾ squat you'll find you get much closer to your normal squatting weights. As before, you can find the weak parts of your squat (it might not just be the bottom) and build the strength there.

1. Set the pins in the rack accordingly to your height and load up the bar with the weight you're going to use.
2. This exercise is usually started from the bottom portion where you start at the bottom of the partial squat and stand up. Get in your squat stance and put your hands at the appropriate distance. But you can also start from the top.
3. A wider stance will allow you much more power in this position, in a short range partial. It also allows a more upright back rather than leaning forwards. In a half or more partial squat, use your normal squat stance.
4. Breathe in and pressurize everything.
5. Push with the legs and come to a standing position.

This is a great exercise to work up to maximal weights in. Be warned that the first time you do it, your spine may not be used to holding that much weight. And that may be part of the T-boosting too. It is recommended to decompress by hanging from a pullup bar between sets.

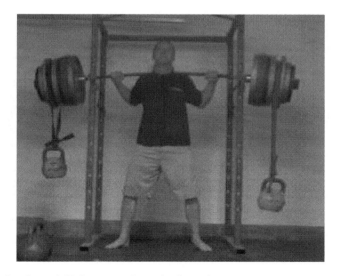

Push Press

When it comes to testosterone boosting, working the lower body is king. Nothing beats the squat and deadlift. But I think you can achieve much of the effect training the upper body as well. My top pick for this, besides the partial I'll cover next, is the push press.

While the military press, or a side press, are good, the push press allows you to handle more weight and use more muscle. The legs get involved. But it is not as technical as the jerk, which would allow you to handle more weight. So because it is user friendly and you can handle a good amount of weight, it is my favorite upper body exercise for this goal. (If you're well practiced in the Olympic jerk, by all means, use that.)

The bench press certainly also works as you can handle very heavy weights but, overall, I think it's more manly to stand and lift then lay down and do so. If muscle building is your goal than the bench press is hard to beat.

This can be done with dumbbells, kettlebells, and odd objects which will be covered later, though the best bet is the barbell for maximal load.

1. Clean the weight into place or take it from a power rack to the shoulders.
2. Dip the legs down about a quarter of the way.
3. Driving with the legs, explode upwards, and pushing with the arms at the same time.
4. Lockout the weight overhead with your whole body aligned.
5. Lower the weight and repeat.

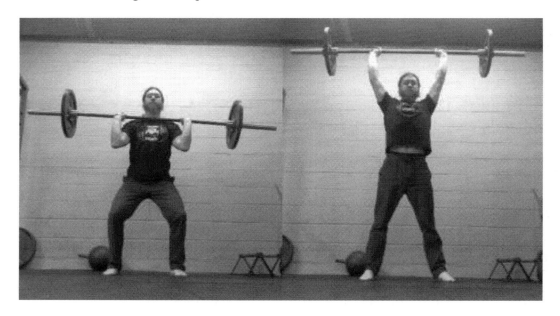

112

Overhead Support

Legendary lifter John Grimek is said to have supported 1000 lbs. overhead. You can't deny that he had strong T going for him, just by looking at him.

Many power racks are not high enough to allow you to lift overhead in this manner. Mine is not, unless I put the barbell on top of the rack. Due to the slight bend in the bars I have due to using very heavy weights for partials and supports there is no danger in it rolling off the rack. Whatever you do make sure you have a stable and safe place to work these. Another option is to hang a barbell from chains off the ceiling as Grimek did. In doing this make sure you're hanging it off of a strong enough load bearing beam!

There are a couple different ways to approach overhead lifting in this manner.

When it comes to the partial lift you want to be sure you're pressing out with your arms. This will build very strong triceps, and the whole body will be working to support them as well. But this will limit the weight you can use. Even with the partial position, the arms and shoulders will be the weak link.

Another option is starting with the arms already locked out and then basically doing a partial overhead squat. The legs are much stronger than the arms and thus you'll be able to handle more weight like this.

Thus, I like to use the legs to get a support into place. With the support the shoulders and triceps will still be working very hard to hold onto the large weight and keep it from coming down. Then the whole body has to work to stabilize in this leveraged out position. Hold for a second or two then come down.

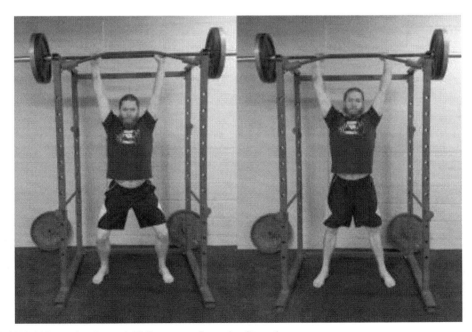

Odd Objects

Rocks, barrels, sandbags, logs and other odd objects are great for lifting. Plus there is something more primal and manlier about lifting an object that isn't made to be lifted. It becomes more of a competition against the object itself.

When I was training for a recent strongman competition I found a few rocks I could lift in my yard. When I first approached them they felt very heavy. But I knew I'd be able to get the smaller of the two overhead in a short amount of time. I could only get it to the shoulders in the first workout, but got it overhead the following one. From there I started repping out with it.

There was also a second, significantly heavier rock. This one I dead lifted and carried. I was also able to shoulder it. My future goal with this would be to put it overhead eventually. You'll see the workout I did with these in the workouts section.

Since you can't easily add or subtract weight, the progression is more about what you can do with them. You compete with the object to be able to handle it better and more so. The same is true with any of the other odd objects.

Of course the main idea of using something heavy holds true here. Lots of gyms carry sandbags these days but they're light. I feel that a 'true' sandbag is something monstrous and difficult to handle, not something you do all kinds of exercises with, just the basics. There is a place for those, but it's different.

The basics, applicable to pretty much all odd objects, include just four exercises:

- Deadlift
- Shoulder
- Overhead
- Carry

The deadlift involves picking the object off the ground, standing up with it, to hip level, and you're done. Note that with many objects you cannot do the classic deadlift form. In fact, with odd object lifting, you often have to take on a round back posture. And that's one of the benefits! The arms and hands often get much more work too.

Shouldering an odd object is just like it sounds. You lift it up to the shoulders like in a clean, or on top of a single shoulder. Sometimes you can clean the weight. But with logs or rocks you often have to set it in your lap, then roll it up. Or do some form of continental. With stones you can roll it over one shoulder, let it drop, and then repeat.

Getting it overhead involves first shouldering then putting it overhead. For something light this can be a military press, but more often than not, you'll be push pressing or jerking it into position.

Carrying can be done in a few different ways. You can carry it by your hips as in the top of the deadlift. You can carry it at your chest or on top of one shoulder. And you can also carry it overhead. So it's just a matter of doing any of the previous three exercises and then starting to walk around with it. Carrying taxes the whole body, including the grip most of the time, as well as engaging your cardiovascular system.

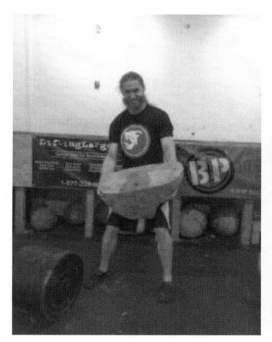
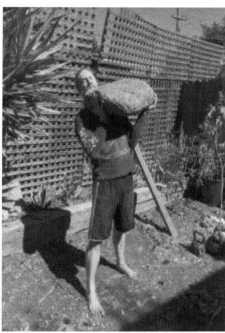

Handstand Pushups

Everything so far has included heavy weights, whether with barbells or odd objects. As described in principle number one of testosterone boosting, I feel this is very important. But it's not the only way. I wanted to give you a couple other options that requires no equipment.

First of all, I recognize that not everyone can do handstand pushups. I certainly could not when I started training. The aim is to work up to handstand pushups and then keep doing them always in more progressive manners. Because you can't just add weight to this exercise, here are a few progressive exercises you can do towards this aim.

- Pushups
- Decline Pushups
- Pike Press
- Steep Decline Pushups
- Handstand Pushups
- Full Range Handstand Pushups

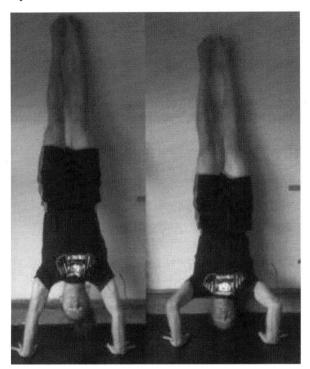

That's not the only way to train this move, and it can take a while to move from one step to the next, but this progression will work. Let me also state that I prefer handstand pushups over one arm pushups because you work both arms at the same time and handle 100% of your bodyweight.

1. Kick up into a handstand against the wall.
2. Keep your head in line with your arms, and bend the elbows to lower yourself under control until your crown touches the floor.
3. Press back up to lockout.

To make this exercise easier lean more into the wall and spread your hands wider. You can also lower down to objects and make the range of motion less. To make it harder maintain a more upright positions and bring the hands even closer.

Depending on where your strength is you may only do a single rep, or you can do more than 10 (though at this point start you should working on the full range version).

Find out much more in The Ultimate Guide to Handstand Pushups at
http://www.legendarystrength.com/products/ultimate-guide-to-handstand-pushups/

Pullups

Once again, I recognize that not everyone can do pullups, though more can do them than the previous exercise. A man must be able to do pullups, just in case you're hanging and your life depends on it. Pullups are easier to add weight to, by attaching weights to a belt, but before you get there, here are a few progressive exercises you can do to work up the main bodyweight exercise.

- Leaning Row
- Inverted Row
- Jumping Chin-up with Negative
- Assisted Chin-up

In general, the chin-up with the palms facing towards you is easier to most people than the pullup, with the palms facing away. But this also depends on how use to each version you are.

Let me also state that lat pulldowns are not the equivalent to real pullups. Skip the machine and work the bodyweight version as best as you can.

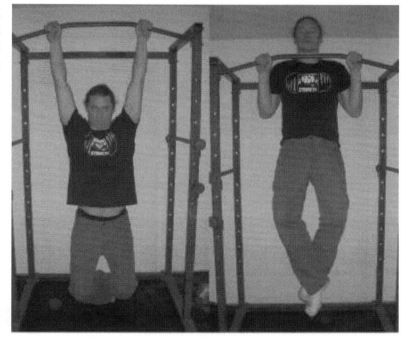

1. Hang from the bar with arms completely locked out.
2. Start the pull by packing in the shoulders.
3. Bend the arms and pull your chin over the bar.
4. Lower fully under control.

Of course once you can do pullups you can start training harder versions like working towards the one arm pullup. As mentioned you can also easily add weight to the regular exercise, which then makes it something you can work at a desired rep range as covered earlier.

Find out much more in The Ultimate Guide to Pullups & Chin-Ups at
http://legendarystrength.com/ultimate-guide-pullups/

Hanging Leg Raises

I believe that the upper and lower body training is more important than focusing on the abs when it comes to testosterone. But I add this exercise here because I typically teach these four bodyweight exercises together. Plus people always want ab training.

This is one of my favorite bodyweight ab exercises. Once again there is a simple progression we can use to get up to this main exercise.

- Floor Leg Raises
- Hanging Knee Raises
- Partial Hanging Leg Raises

As for the regular exercise, here are the steps.

1. Start hanging from the bar.
2. Keeping the knees locked out, raise the legs until they are parallel with the ground. The toes ankle can be bent (as pictured below) or the toes can be pointed. Your body should look like an L when seen from the side.
3. Lower under control.

If this exercise is easy, you can work towards full hanging leg raises where the legs touch the bar. You can also use ankle weights to make it much tougher to do.

Find out much more in The Ultimate Guide to Bodyweight Ab Exercises at
http://legendarystrength.com/ultimate-guide-abs/

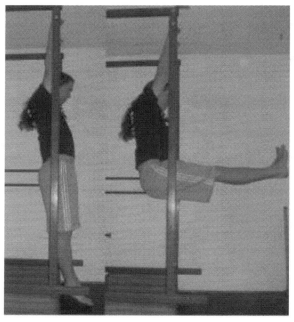

One Legged Squats

The regular squat basically involves all the muscles of the legs. It's a simple exercise and a general movement pattern that everyone should have. If you can't you'll want to train this movement so that you can squat rock bottom. It's not necessary for good testosterone, but it's necessary for good movement quality.

For T purposes, when sticking to bodyweight exercises, you'll want to move beyond that towards the one leg versions. This does take more flexibility to do, but is a worthy goal for most. To build up to it:

- Regular Squats
- Legs Together Squats
- Partial One Legged Squat

Here is how you do a one legged pistol squat.

1. Stand on one leg with your weight centered over it. The opposite leg will be held out to the front.
2. Squat back and down, leaning forward to counterbalance your weight. To reach the bottom position you need to lean far forward and you also need some active flexibility to keep the free leg off of the ground.
3. Press hard into the ground and come up to a standing position.

Once you've achieved this exercise you can start to add weight. (Using a small counterweight is another option for helping you achieve this movement, as it actually makes it easier to do.)

Find out much more in The Ultimate Guide to Bodyweight Squats and Pistols at http://legendarystrength.com/ultimate-guide-squats/

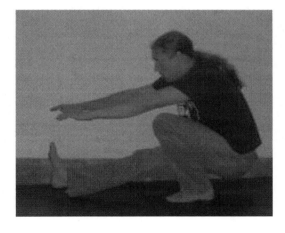

Animal Movements

Remember that *animalistic* was one of the *feelings of testosterone*, and there's no better way to get into that feeling than to move like an animal. While there are tons of variations, here are my two favorites for this purpose:

Bear Crawl - Your hands and feet are on the floor with your butt up in the air. This position allows you to move pretty fast, but it can also be effective (and possibly even harder) to move slowly.

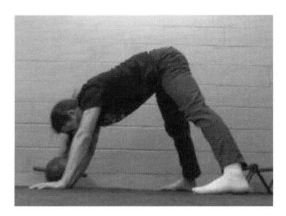

Ape - Start with your hands and feet on the floor. This time your knees are bent so your back is roughly parallel to the floor. You can also be on your fists rather than with the palms flat on the floor. Shoot forward with both of your hands at the same time, then bring both of your legs between them. Continue moving in this manner both hands at once, then both legs at once. Grunting and making ape noises is optional. It takes some coordination to do this movement, but once you have the hang of it you can move quite quickly.

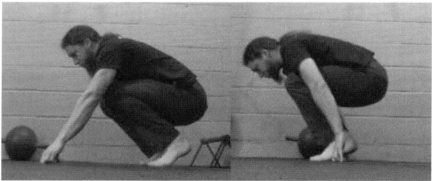

Generally, when working with these, pick a distance and a number of times to go. For much more about animal movements and how to use them I suggest you check out my buddy, Mike Fitch, and his Animal Flow program. In addition to the basic movements it covers a lot more of unique and novel ways to use them. Not necessarily the best for T, but awesome nonetheless. http://www.legendarystrength.com/go/animal/

Hill Sprints

While I think of hill sprints as more of a growth hormone releasing exercise, they certainly boost testosterone as well. And while I'll only address hill sprints here, since they're my favorite, and what I believe to be most effective, you can get much of the same benefits by stair sprinting or flat land sprints.

Hill sprints shouldn't be something you jump into right away, depending on your current conditioning level. Instead, it is wise to ease into it. Every time I go back to them, when I haven't done them in some time, I don't go all out on my first session. I run the hills, but I don't do all out sprints. This helps limit the soreness they can bring too. (My shins always get sore the first time I do them after a layoff.)

For those not in great shape already, jogging may be all you can muster. Even for sedentary folks just walking the hill may be the most optimal choice. Ease into this intense exercise. The good news is that running on hills is actually safer than running on flat ground.

The ideal hill will have a decent slope and a length of what you can sprint in about 30 seconds. If you go longer than 30 seconds you'll typically find you can't keep an all-out pace. It's great to mix it up every once in a while, but this is the optimal explosive hill sprint distance. Of course, the steeper the incline the harder it will be to do.

In all your training you must keep it progressive. This way you know you are doing better. For this reason you should run the same length most of the time. Have a start and a finish line. And time yourself for each sprint. Race yourself trying to beat your best time each and every time. It is satisfying to see over the course of a couple weeks how what took you 30 seconds before now only takes you 27.

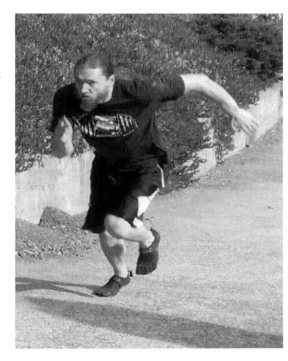

For every single step you want to go faster. This gets you out of breath quick. With many other conditioning exercises there is time in the move to relax, even if just for a split second. Even going at a fast pace it's really not all out like hill sprints can be at every moment. With a steep hill you will get out of breath fast.

Example Workouts

When it comes to testosterone, and increasing it, it's something we want to do each day. As these are mostly short workouts, not meant to be catabolic in nature, you can do this work each day. A single set of squats done daily, will likely do more for your hormones, than a harder squat workout once a week.

Since the training is not done to failure, or for high volume, it's not going to break down tissue as much as other training does, leaving you sore and in need of several days to recuperate.

The goal is to be successful, so even though it's "heavy" it doesn't have to be a maximum each day. In fact it shouldn't. That could drain the nervous system, even if your muscles were fresh. As that is a form of fatigue, which can lead to overtraining, it's to be avoided, or at least limited, as well.

But each exercise doesn't have to be done every day either. You can alternate and mix them up. The important thing would be to do some form of training four to six days a week. And I'd lean towards more. You could go seven but I think at least one day off a week is a good protocol to follow.

As for the workout itself there are many ways to do it. The following are a few different workout schedules and individual workouts. While you can use these as is, I advise making anything your own. Use them as starting templates and then individualize. Use them to generate your own ideas to make them work best for you.

The 5x5 T-Boosting Schedule

The 5 sets of 5 workout is a classic and it can work well for this purpose. Depending on the weights it can be fatiguing though, so be sure to keep it easy enough, while still progressing.

The best way to do it is with the first and second sets as warm-ups. Then the final three sets are with your working weight. If you hit five reps on all three of these sets, then you'll increase the weight you use next time.

Take two to five minutes of rest per set. The warmups can be done quicker. All in all each workout will take about 15-25 minutes.

This can be applied to any of our three main T-boosting exercises, deadlifts, squats and push presses. It would also work for partials. A six day a week schedule could include both.

Monday - 5x5 Deadlift
Tuesday - 5x5 Push Press
Wednesday - 5x5 Squat
Thursday - 5x5 Rack Pull
Friday - 5x5 Overhead Lockout
Saturday - 5x5 Partial Squat
Sunday - Rest

If you can't train each day you could mix and match these in a few different ways.

Monday - 5x5 Deadlift and 5x5 Overhead Lockout
Tuesday - Rest
Wednesday - 5x5 Push Press and 5x5 Partial Squat
Thursday - Rest
Friday - 5x5 Squat and 5x5 Rack Pull
Saturday - Variety Day
Sunday - Rest

Remember to start with a moderately heavy weight to ensure your success. Then increase little by little.

The 3x3 T-Boosting Schedule

Three sets of three allows you to use a bit heavier of a weight, for less volume. For some people this will work better than the 5x5.

In this one, warm-up sets don't count, so once again you could do one or two of these, then the three sets of three are your working sets.

Other than that, everything is the same as the 5x5.

Another similar option would be 5/3/1.

Rest Pause Training

Rest pause training is a different way of doing reps in a given set. Instead of doing each rep right after another, back to back, without stopping, here you pause. After each rep you stop for a breath or a few and then go again.

In squats you stand at the top as you rest, still supporting the weight. In deadlifts you rest with the bar on the floor, usually still holding onto it. In the push press you hold the weight in the clean or rack position. With an odd object you'll generally release it on the ground. In partials, it's usually supported by the rack.

You can do the 5x5 or 3x3 schedules using rest pause training.

Another option is a single working set of 8-10 reps. This is higher reps per set than normally recommended, but with rest-pause style, it's kind of like doing a series of heavy singles. The weight is heavy, but not so heavy, that you can't handle it for this single set. Here's an example of how that could be put together.

Monday - 1x10 Rest-Pause Deadlift
Tuesday - 1x10 Rest-Pause Push Press
Wednesday - 1x10 Rest-Pause Squat
Thursday - 1x10 Rest-Pause Rack Pull
Friday - 1x10 Rest-Pause Overhead Lockout
Saturday - 1x10 Rest-Pause Partial Squat
Sunday - Rest

Some type of warmup would be advised before getting to this set. But besides that, a single set of training each day could do a lot for you.

Heavy Singles Up to a Max with Variation

In this workout, you're working up to a max for the day. While it is ideal if it is an all-time max, this probably won't be the case every day, at least not for the main lifts. But this can be better achieved if you include lots of variations of the exercises, as described in the variations of each exercise, or different partial ranges. The benefit of doing so is that when working with lots of things you can set lots of different PR's. By being successful you release more T.

Warm-up as needed then start doing singles with progressively heavier weights until you get to your best for the day. Remember, to ensure you're successful. It's best to stop when you feel like you could do more. Far better to do so, leaving some in the tank, than to fail on a set.

I like to use the signals from my body as far as what feels best to do in a given day. While squatting may feel good, front squats may feel better. Although front squats mean a lighter weight, I'll listen to my body instead of forcing it in one direction whenever possible.

You could do a couple different lifts in a given workout. Below is an example of two for each workout, spread out over five days a week. Once again, this is just an example, so don't take it as gospel.

Monday - Up to Heavy Single Sumo Deadlift and Up to Heavy Single Overhead Lockout
Tuesday - Up to Heavy Single Zercher Squat and Up to Heavy Single Push Press
Wednesday - Up to Heavy Single Jefferson Deadlift and Up to Heavy Single Half Squat
Thursday - Rest
Friday - Up to Heavy Single Short Rack Pull and Up to Heavy Single Bench Press
Saturday - Up to Heavy Single ¾ Deadlift and Up to Heavy Single Front Squat
Sunday - Rest

Heavy Partials Reverse Pyramid

This is similar to the above, but how I specifically like to approach partials. Since it's a shorter range of motion, I feel a bit more volume can be handled, especially if it's a short range partial.

First select the partial you're going to work on for the given day. Start with a light weight and do 20-30 reps with this. Add weight and do 10-15 reps. More weight and less reps. More weight and less reps again. Finally you'll get to doing singles and you can keep doing more weight, continuing until you get to a heavy max single for the day.

By using different ranges of motion, on different days, the same as with the variations as previously mentioned, you can manage lots of different PR's with singles here.

Several Times a Day Training

This has also been called Grease the Groove training (GTG), as popularized by Pavel Tsatsouline. While the principle idea in that was to practice strength as a skill, here it can be applied to boosting testosterone several times a day.

If lifting a heavy weight increases testosterone in the moment and for some time afterwards, what would occur if you did that ten times in a day? You'd have lots of T spikes which probably will generalize into higher testosterone on a general basis.

The exercise selection here are not high skill movements. In fact, they're some of the lowest skill exercises out there (not to say skill isn't involved at all). Instead we use a moderately heavy weight, working multiple times a day. This can be from 5 to 15 times. The important thing once again, is to not get fatigued or to struggle. If it is becoming hard at the end of the day, chances are the weight is too heavy.

The weight should also be light enough that you can do it "from cold," that is without a warm-up. Though it should also still be heavy enough to get the desired effect. Because they're easier to do cold, partials can also be used for this purpose.

I like singles, doubles and triples for this, but you could go as high as five. Just be aware as the reps go up, the total sets per day should go down. Otherwise you can end up with too much total volume and thus fatigue. Here's one example mixing up the exercises as before.

Monday - 5-15 Times a Day Deadlift x 1-5
Tuesday - 5-15 Times a Day Push Press x 1-5
Wednesday - 5-15 Times a Day Squat x 1-5
Thursday - 5-15 Times a Day Rack Pull x 1-5
Friday - 5-15 Times a Day Overhead Lockout x 1-5
Saturday - 5-15 Times a Day Partial Squat x 1-5
Sunday - Rest

The only way to really do this is to have the weights setup and ready to go in a location not far from where you'll be on a daily basis. If this isn't feasible for you, then this may not be the best training schedule for you.

With this schedule you could also stick to just two exercises and do them daily. Watch that you don't become sore or fatigued as the week goes on. If you do, take an extra day or two off and/or reduce the load or volume a bit. Below I've chosen the deadlift and push press but you could use any two exercises. Probably an upper and lower body would be best. Do both of these exercises together after a little bit of rest.

The great thing about this schedule besides helping to boost testosterone all day long, is that it doesn't take any dedicated time. If it is feasible for you it just takes a minute or two several times a day and nothing more.

Monday - 5-15 Times a Day Deadlift x 1-5 and Push Press x 1-5
Tuesday - 5-15 Times a Day Deadlift x 1-5 and Push Press x 1-5
Wednesday - 5-15 Times a Day Deadlift x 1-5 and Push Press x 1-5
Thursday - 5-15 Times a Day Deadlift x 1-5 and Push Press x 1-5
Friday - 5-15 Times a Day Deadlift x 1-5 and Push Press x 1-5
Saturday - 5-15 Times a Day Deadlift x 1-5 and Push Press x 1-5
Sunday - Rest

Odd Object Challenge

Pick one to three odd objects. These can be of the same type, like different size rocks, or different objects. What you'll do with these depends on the size and weight of the object. If you can only deadlift it you'll do that. If you can shoulder it you'll do that. If you can get it overhead you'll do that. And you can add a carry of any type to anyone of these.

The recommended rep ranges are from a single to twelve reps. Sometimes you'll have to go higher than the earlier recommendation of under five just because of what the weight of the object is.

If using a single object, take sufficient rest between sets. If using multiple objects go back and forth between them in a circuit fashion, but once again take sufficient rest.

A recent stone lifting workout that I was doing, involving two stones, looked like this.

1) Clean and put overhead as many times as I could (started out with singles and eventually worked up to eight reps) the smaller rock.

2) Shoulder the bigger rock x 1.

3) Deadlift and carry for distance the bigger rock.

I repeated this for about three to six rounds and was finished. It probably took about 20 minutes.

Big Four Bodyweight Workouts

The following workout can be done up to three times per week, assuming you properly recover from it. It is best done in a circuit fashion, going from one exercise to the next but with adequate rest so that you're recovered.

If you can't do each exercise, do any of the easier variations, and change up sets and reps as you see fit.

HSPU x 5-10 sets x 3-10 reps
Pullups x 5-10 sets x 3-10 reps
One-Legged Squats x 5-10 sets x 3-10 reps each leg
Hanging Leg Raises x 5-10 sets x 3-10 reps

This could also be split up on different days and then done six times per week like so:

Monday - HSPU and Pullups x 5-10 sets x 3-10 reps each
Tuesday - One-Legged Squats and Hanging Leg Raises x 5-10 sets x 3-10 reps each
Wednesday - HSPU and Pullups x 5-10 sets x 3-10 reps each
Thursday - One-Legged Squats and Hanging Leg Raises x 5-10 sets x 3-10 reps each
Friday - HSPU and Pullups x 5-10 sets x 3-10 reps each
Saturday - One-Legged Squats and Hanging Leg Raises x 5-10 sets x 3-10 reps each
Sunday – Rest

If you wanted to work some weights and some bodyweight it could be the following:

Monday – Barbell Squats 5x5
Tuesday – HSPU and Pullups x 5-10 sets x 3-10 reps each
Wednesday – Rest
Thursday – Deadlifts 5x5
Friday – HSPU and Pullups x 5-10 sets x 3-10 reps each
Saturday – Hill Sprints x 4-8
Sunday – Rest

Hill Sprint Workout

I find that four to eight sprints is enough for the workout, and that takes some building up to. You know you are in condition when your last sprint is not more than a second or two in time off of the first. But when you're starting out don't be surprised to find yourself taking five to eight seconds longer on that last sprint. And if that's the case you probably should have stopped earlier as now you're fatigued.

After you finish the sprint walk down to the bottom and start again. Your only rest is in the walk down. This same style works even if you're starting out walking or jogging up the hill. It's the natural interval built into hill running. Of course, in the beginning if you need more time to recover, rest at the bottom of the hill.

Typically hill sprints are done two or three times a week, depending on other leg training and conditioning exercise. Doing hill sprints a couple times a week will make you tougher, better conditioned, stronger, and faster. Well worth the effort.

Animalistic Playing

Select a distance, and travel across it in one animal, and come back as a different animal. Repeat this for a set number of times. Take short breaks between each round.

Bear Crawl x 50 m
Ape x 50 m
Repeat 5-10 times

This can be done two to three times a week like the hill sprint workout, since it is much like sprinting. But the upper body is involved quite a bit more in these so you may need to modify other training. Great to add in one session as a variety day where needed.

Mixed Training

You can mix and match from the above as well. Here's a 4 day a week schedule.

Monday - Hill Sprints
Tuesday - Rest
Wednesday - 5x5 Push Press and 5x5 Squat
Thursday - Rest
Friday - Odd Object Lifting
Saturday - 5x5 Deadlifts, HSPU and Pullups
Sunday - Rest

The Science of T-Boosting Workouts

What is shown in this book is mostly my experience of what can and will boost testosterone. Not everything suggested or theorized is backed by science. While I would love to have some of these ideas put to the test in a research study, some of them are too far outside the conventional training world (like doing partials it seems), that it will likely not happen at least for many years. Personally, I'm not going to wait for that before training like this.

I dug through research to see what was "proven" about boosting T. I put the word proven in quotes because there are oftentimes contradictory results, and not every study is as high quality as others. Plus with small sample sizes, and specific population groups used, it doesn't necessarily mean that what worked in the studies would work for you. Ideal science is in a "closed system" but basically that's impossible to really achieve. And science doesn't actually prove anything, it just helps establish a theory. There are lots of confounding influences that can lead to different results.

In addition to pulling quotes from these studies, I'll add my commentary about each one. If you don't want your eyes to glaze over reading the short quote, typically from the abstract of the study, I also summarize what the research means. Some of these are in alignment with what I've established in the rest of this guide, while some are not, and I detail on why that may be the case as such.

From a report titled:
Differential effects of strength training leading to failure versus not to failure on hormonal responses, strength, and muscle power gains. [1]
"The purpose of this study was to examine the efficacy of 11 wk of resistance training to failure vs. no failure...Forty-two physically active men were matched and then randomly assigned to either a training to failure (RF; n = 14), nonfailure (NRF; n = 15), or control groups (C; n = 13)...NRF resulted in reduced resting cortisol concentrations and an elevation in resting serum total testosterone concentration."

My summary and commentary:
This showed that not going to failure increased resting testosterone levels more than going to failure. The resting testosterone is interesting, because while many exercises seem to spike testosterone for a time after the training, this showed an increase in regular levels. It's not surprising to me that cortisol went down, because it's less stressful to not go to failure. This backs up my second principle.

From a report titled:
Hormonal responses of multiset versus single-set heavy-resistance exercise protocols. [2]
"The purpose of this study was to compare serum growth hormone (GH), testosterone (T), cortisol (C), and whole blood lactate (L) responses to single set (1S) versus multiple set (3S) heavy-resistance exercise protocols. Eight recreationally weight-trained men completed two identical resistance exercise workouts (1S vs. 3S). Blood was obtained

preexercise (PRE), immediately postexercise (OP), and 5 min (5P), 15 min (15P), 30 min (30P) and 60 min (60P) postexercise and was analyzed for GH, T, C, and L levels. For 1S and 3S, GH, L, and T significantly increased from PRE to OP and remained significantly elevated to 60P, except for 1S. For GH, T, and L, 3S showed significantly greater increases compared to 1S."

My summary and commentary:
This research indicates that three sets of an exercise outperformed doing a single set. While both increased T, the three sets kept it higher longer and was significantly higher. While I advocated low volume it's generally not that low. More than one set has been typically recommended.

From a report titled:
Effects of very short rest periods on hormonal responses to resistance exercise in men. [3]
"The effect of 3 different rest periods on the acute hormonal responses to resistance exercise (RE) was examined in 10 experienced resistance trained men ... subjects were assigned in a random order a rest interval of 60 seconds (P60), 90 seconds (P90), or 120 seconds (P120) between sets...Serum TS concentrations were significantly higher at T1 in P120 (65%) and P90 (76%) compared to P60 (p < or = 0.05)...TS response was greater in the RE protocol with a 120-second rest interval between sets."

My summary and commentary:
This report shows a best response in boosting testosterone by resting 2 minutes between sets, compared to one minute, or a minute and a half. I personally would like to have seen a broader range tested, though you do see that in a later study. And this exercise was a bench press done to failure. But this does show that a rest enough to bring back most of your strength is best.

From a report titled:
Order effects of combined strength and endurance training on testosterone, cortisol, growth hormone and IGFBP-3 in concurrent-trained men. [4]
"The aim of this study was to compare the acute effects of two different orders of concurrent training on hormonal responses in concurrent trained men. Fourteen men were randomly divided into 2 groups: endurance training followed by strength and strength training followed by endurance. Serum concentrations of testosterone, cortisol, growth hormone and IGFBP3 were measured before and after both training orders...The testosterone and IGFBP-3 concentrations significantly increased in the ES group after the exercise trainings, but did not change significantly in the SE group... In conclusion, these results suggest that immediately post-exercise testosterone and IGFPB-3 responses are significantly increased only after the ES order. Therefore, an ES training order should be prescribed if the main focus of the training intervention is to induce an acute post-exercise anabolic environment."

My summary and commentary:
Only the endurance followed by strength group saw an increase in testosterone, while the

strength followed by endurance did not. The latter is the generally recommended training format. My guess is that doing endurance after strength "kills" the testosterone increase as cortisol probably goes up. But if you do endurance first, then strength, you see the boost still. So if testosterone is your goal it would be wise to limit your endurance work, or do it first. Plus the endurance training was running on a treadmill, and I wouldn't recommend that.

From a report titled:
Acute hormonal responses to heavy resistance exercise in strength athletes versus nonathletes. [5]
"The aim of the present study was to investigate acute hormonal and neuromuscular responses and recovery in strength athletes versus nonathletes during heavy resistance exercise performed with the forced and maximum repetitions training protocol. Eight male strength athletes (SA) with several years of continuous resistance training experience and 8 physically active but non-strength athletes (NA) volunteered as subjects. The experimental design comprised two loading sessions: maximum repetitions (MR) and forced repetitions (FR)... These data suggest that, at least in experienced strength athletes, the forced-repetition protocol is a viable alternative to the more traditional maximum-repetition protocol and may even be a superior approach."

My summary and commentary:
In this study going beyond failure boosted testosterone more than going to failure. It would have been interesting to see a non-training to failure group in this one, as we saw that earlier outperform training to failure. That being said, I do believe that every once in a while you do want to push yourself to the edge and even beyond it. It's manly to do so. You just can't do it so often that it burns you out. So every once in a while go very hard, but regularly I still recommend not going to failure.

From a report titled:
The Acute Hormonal Response to Free Weight and Machine Weight Resistance Exercise [6]
"The purpose of this study was to examine the effect of resistance exercise selection on the acute hormonal response using similar lower-body multijoint movement free weight and machine weight exercises...Exercise increased (p = 0.05) T and GH at IP, but the concentrations at IP were greater for the squat than for the leg press...Free weight exercises seem to induce greater hormonal responses to resistance exercise than machine weight exercises using similar lower-body multijoint movements and primary movers."

My summary and commentary:
For any real lifter these results aren't surprising. A barbell squat outperformed a machine leg press in boosting testosterone and other hormones. Why this is isn't known, but it's hypothesized to do with the load being more on the body with the squat than the leg press. It may also have to do with more stabilization coming into effect. If the latter is the case, I'd be very curious in how an odd object, or partial squat, might compare and possibly outperform even the full range squat.

From a report titled:

Age-independent increases in male salivary testosterone during horticultural activity among Tsimane forager-farmers. [7]

"This study examines acute changes in salivary testosterone among 63 Tsimane men ranging in age from 16–80 years during one-hour bouts of tree-chopping while clearing horticultural plots... A comparison of these results to the relative change in testosterone during a competitive soccer tournament in the same population reveals larger relative changes in testosterone following resource production (tree chopping), compared to competition (soccer)."

My summary and commentary:

This is an interesting one. It showed that chopping wood, a manly activity, for an hour boosted testosterone 48.6%, much better than a competitive soccer game. Although that's not a specific training protocol, to me, it helps point in the direction of odd object training. It would be interesting to compare that to weightlifting.

From a report titled:

Anabolic processes in human skeletal muscle: restoring the identities of growth hormone and testosterone. [8]

"There is a persistent belief (both in scientific literature and among recreational weightlifters) that exercise-induced release of GH and testosterone underpins muscular hypertrophy with resistance training... Our recent work disputes this assumption... Data from our training study demonstrate that exercise-induced increases in GH and testosterone availability are not necessary for and do not enhance strength and hypertrophy adaptations.... Clarifying both the role of hormones in regulating muscle mass as well as the underlying basis for adaptation of skeletal muscle to resistance exercise will hopefully enhance and support the prescription of resistance exercise as an integral component of a healthy lifestyle."

My summary and commentary:

Although testosterone and growth hormone are correlated to muscle mass, in that in the elderly that loss of testosterone results in sarcopenia, the inverse may not be true. The elevations in anabolic hormones by training may not be the responsible part for increasing muscle or strength. Of course, strength can come through multiple ways. But this doesn't refute that you can increase your testosterone, for the other effects, through exercise.

From a report titled:

The acute hormonal response to the kettlebell swing exercise. [9]

"The purpose of this investigation was to examine the acute hormonal response to the kettlebell swing exercise. Ten recreationally resistance trained men performed 12 rounds of 30 seconds of 16 kg kettlebell swings alternated with 30 seconds of rest... Testosterone was significantly higher (p = 0.05) at IP than at PRE, P15, or P30... The exercise protocol produced an acute increase in hormones involved in muscle adaptations. Thus, the

kettlebell swing exercise might provide a good supplement to resistance training programs."

My summary and commentary:
I just had to include the study on the kettlebell when I saw it. This showed that kettlebell swings increased testosterone right after the exercise, but that this increase did not continue. It would be interesting to see if a heavier load, and less of a conditioning based protocol, would cause a bigger or longer lasting release.

From a report titled:
Resistance training restores muscle sex steroid hormone steroidogenesis in older men. [10]
"Skeletal muscle can synthesize testosterone and 5α-dihydrotestosterone (DHT) from dehydroepiandrosterone (DHEA) via steroidogenic enzymes in vitro, but hormone levels and steroidogenic enzyme expression decline with aging. Resistance exercise has been shown to increase in plasma sex steroid hormone levels...Six young and 13 older men were recruited...Muscular sex steroid hormone levels and sex steroidgenesis-related enzyme expressions were significantly lower in older subjects than younger ones at baseline, but 12 wk of resistance training significantly restored hormone levels...We conclude progressive resistance training restores age-related declines in sex steroidogenic enzyme and muscle sex steroid hormone levels in older men."

My summary and commentary:
This studied showed that resistance training was effective in restoring the hormone levels of older men. It doesn't matter your age, you can get better.

From a report titled:
Salivary testosterone is related to self-selected training load in elite female athletes. [11]
"It is our contention that testosterone may also contribute to improved volitional motivation and, when monitored longitudinally, may provide one proxy marker for readiness to perform. Twelve female netball players provided saliva samples prior to five standardized training sessions in which they completed a maximal-distance medicine ball throw, and then 3 sets of bench press and then back squat using a self-selected load perceived to equal a 3-repetition maximum load. Additional repetitions were encouraged when possible...Individual salivary testosterone, when viewed relatively over time, demonstrated strong relationships with self-selected workloads during an in-season training period in female netball players. As such, daily variations in testosterone may provide information regarding voluntary training motivation and readiness to perform in elite athletic populations. Psychological and behavioral aspects of testosterone may have the potential to enhance training adaptation by complementing the known anabolic and permissive properties of testosterone."

My summary and commentary:
Although this was with women I thought the idea behind the study was interesting. Rather than looking at whether the exercises boosted testosterone they were correlating

them to performance and motivation via the self-selection of weights. This sounds like the basics of intuitive training to me. It demonstrates the need to modulate workloads based on where your testosterone may be at. I'd be willing to bet similar results would occur in men too.

From a report titled:
Effects of strongman training on salivary testosterone levels in a sample of trained men. [12]

"Strongman exercises consist of multi-joint movements that incorporate large muscle mass groups and impose a substantial amount of neuromuscular stress. The purpose of this study was to examine salivary testosterone responses from 2 novel strongman training (ST) protocols in comparison with an established hypertrophic (H) protocol reported to acutely elevate testosterone levels. Sixteen men (24 ± 4.4 years, 181.2 ± 6.8 cm, and 95.3 ± 20.3 kg) volunteered to participate in this study. Subjects completed 3 protocols designed to ensure equal total volume (sets and repetitions), rest period, and intensity between the groups. Exercise sets were performed to failure. Exercise selection and intensity (3 sets × 10 repetitions at 75% 1 repetition maximum) were chosen as they reflected commonly prescribed resistance exercise protocols recognized to elicit a large acute hormonal response. In each of the protocols, subjects were required to perform 3 sets to muscle failure of 5 different exercises (tire flip, chain drag, farmers walk, keg carry, and atlas stone lift) with a 2-minute rest interval between sets and a 3-minute rest interval between exercises. Saliva samples were collected pre-exercise (PRE), immediate postexercise (PST), and 30 minutes postexercise (30PST). Delta scores indicated a significant difference between PRE and PST testosterone level within each group (p = 0.05), with no significant difference between the groups. Testosterone levels spiked 136% (225.23 ± 148.01 pg·ml(-1)) for the H group, 74% (132.04 ± 98.09 pg·ml(-1)) for the ST group, and 54% (122.10 ± 140.67 pg·ml) for the mixed strongman/hypertrophy (XST) group. A significant difference for testosterone level occurred over time (PST to 30PST) for the H group p = 0.05. In conclusion, ST elicits an acute endocrine response similar to a recognized H protocol when equated for duration and exercise intensity."

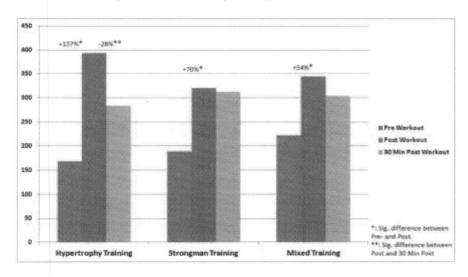

My summary and commentary:
So here we actually see some odd object lifting tested in the form of strongman training. Both the hypertrophy and the strongman protocol boosted testosterone, though the hypertrophy protocol did more so right after the exercise. Though not statistically significant, we see a slightly higher amount of testosterone 30 minutes after training in both the strongman and mixed trainings, over hypertrophy. What I would like to see is some different training formats. Going to failure in strongman exercises, which are largely more full body in each one than in the other exercises used could contribute to too much fatigue which would limit testosterone increases in my opinion.

From a report titled:
Short vs. long rest period between the sets in hypertrophic resistance training: influence on muscle strength, size, and hormonal adaptations in trained men. [13]
"The experimental design comprised a 6-month hypertrophic strength-training period including 2 separate 3-month training periods with the crossover design, a training protocol of short rest (SR, 2 minutes) as compared with long rest (LR, 5 minutes) between the sets. ...Both protocols before the experimental training period (month 0) led to large acute increases (p < 0.05-0.001) in serum T, FT, C , and GH concentrations, as well as to large acute decreases (p < 0.05-0.001) in maximal isometric force and EMG activity. However, no significant differences were observed between the protocols...The present study indicated that, within typical hypertrophic strength-training protocols used in the present study, the length of the recovery times between the sets (2 vs. 5 minutes) did not have an influence on the magnitude of acute hormonal and neuromuscular responses or long-term training adaptations in muscle strength and mass in previously strength-trained men."

My summary and commentary:
This research shows no difference between resting two minutes and five minutes between sets. So it appears as long as you get sufficient rest, meaning at least two minutes, you'll be best set to boost testosterone. Recall that earlier, two minutes outperformed one and one and a half.

Appendix: 5 Step Testosterone Jump Start

In my studies of hormones one thing becomes very apparent.

Whether good or bad, these things tend to perpetuate themselves. In fact, this extends to all areas of health and even more, beyond hormones.

All hormones work in the body via feedback loops.

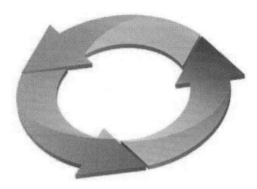

Ideally, what this means is that if something is too low, say testosterone for example, the body takes that feedback, and then will trigger the creation of more.

If it is too high then production will be stopped, or it will be converted or removed, in order to bring it down to normal.

As I said this would be ideal.

However, you'll often get trapped in a cycle of too much or too little of certain hormones. Unfortunately, in those cases, other interactions in the body work to keep you there.

It's like the feedback loops get reset for a less than optimal baseline.

Let's take the example of estrogen dominance. One thing this leads to is the creation of more adipose tissue, i.e. fat. Fat then creates the aromatase enzyme, which converts testosterone into estrogen. The vicious cycle continues…

Another example is with cortisol, the stress hormone. Get too stressed and it becomes harder to relax, throws you sleep off, prevents recovery, and disrupts pretty much all the other hormones too. This in turn leads to more stress and thus more cortisol. Testosterone goes down. The vicious cycle continues…

Not getting enough growth hormone and you'll feel the need for sleep decrease (notice many of the elderly sleep less and less). But what is the biggest trigger of growth hormone? Sleep! The vicious cycle continues…

Your goal is to steer clear of these vicious cycles as best as possible.

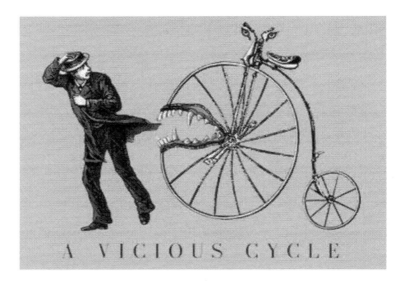

It's not just hormones either. When a person begins to suffer from a chronic disease, if you take the right actions, it can often times be reversed. But at a certain point they become too far gone whether its cancer, heart disease or diabetes. The cycle has continued too long and you can't get out of it.

But there is good news!

The opposite is also true. This is called the "Virtuous Cycle".

This means that the better things are, in general, it is easier to keep them that way.

When you have optimal levels of testosterone you're more likely to be happy. You're more likely to have sex. You're more likely to do some sort of physical activity including workouts.

Guess what? All of these things support testosterone production too!

Hormones are a two-way street. As chemical messengers they both accept messages and relay them. Testosterone may be increased by something…and that something also increases testosterone. This is true when we look at our attitude and the behaviors we engaged in.

When you're entire HPA axis and HPG axis are not off kilter, but are "balanced" and running well, you're better able to take charge of your life and make it even better.

It's much easier to take the time to meditate when you're not stressed the f*ck out!

Eating right helps you to be more active. And being more active helps you to eat right.

With youth, everything is running well typically, and when the "shit hits the fan" you bounce right back. You ever watch a kid take a nasty spill and just get right back up uninjured as if nothing had happened?

They're operating in a virtuous cycle that keeps the status quo of things running well.

But over time…not from the time itself necessarily, but what occurs during it (as Peter Ragnar, a great model of vitality into old age says *"Time is not toxic"*), the cycle slows and eventually can become vicious.

Here, when it hits the fan, you drop deeper into a hole.

A hole that can take years to "dig" yourself out of.

Just like being in debt typically becomes more and more debt. (And the flip side, the virtuous cycle, of wealth becoming more wealth, is also true.)

But even if you're stuck in a vicious cycle, all is not lost. What does it take to move from vicious to virtuous?

Often times it takes massive action. A jumpstart can help get you there. If you are here I highly encourage you to make some big changes.

And that's one of the reasons I love super herbs and select nutrients. They can act as that jumpstart in a way that is simple enough for people to get started.

With the benefits they bring you're better able to make lifestyle changes to support you getting into a virtuous cycle. With testosterone running you'll be better at training, eating right and all the other things you should be doing.

The five-step jumpstart program outlined here is designed to be easy to do and launch you into orbit like a rocket ship.

First of all testosterone production doesn't occur without many vitamins and minerals. There are some very notable ones like zinc and vitamin D, but basically every vitamin and most minerals play a role in the hormonal cascade.

Every single hormone conversion, of which there are many, requires these as co-factors. Thus a single deficiency can throw the whole thing off. No zinc, no testosterone. No potassium and your luteinizing hormone, which triggers the testes to make T is off. No vitamin E and lower testosterone, LH and FSH levels. And on and on it goes.

We are deficient in many things for several reasons. One is that our food, even natural and organic food, often has less because the soil is depleted. If it's not there then it can't be in the plant or the animal. And if you're eating processed food it's even further stripped.

Secondly, with the environmental stressors our bodies actually use up even more of these nutrients than our ancestors did. If you engage in hard training of any type that also means you need more.

So what do you do about it? The simplest solution is to make sure you are on a well-rounded multi-vitamin and mineral supplement. Unfortunately, they are not all created equal, not by a long shot. If you think you're getting covered by any of the popular one-a-day multivitamin, the truth is many of those may be doing more harm than good.

I'm all about getting what you need from real food. Yet I recognize that even eating the highest quality food and taking various herbs may still leave you with gaps when it comes to these nutrients. You'd have to be extremely careful and exact to get everything you really need for optimal functioning.

Thus for many people the best bet is to **make sure you have micronutrient insurance**. For much more on this subject make sure to check out this interview with Jayson and Mira Calton, leaders in this field. https://supermanherbs.com/ep28-micronutrients/

In my opinion, from talking to them and extensively looking at what is available on the market, Nutrience is the best available multivitamin and mineral supplement of this nature. http://legendarystrength.com/go/multivitamin

Furthermore, beyond hormones, it is various chronic micronutrient deficiencies that are root causes of all lifestyle diseases. And once you have your bases covered then you're in a better place to take advantage of super herbs that can assist in hormone production.

While the herbs that I'm about to mention, especially the first one, is loaded with micronutrients itself, it still doesn't have everything in the amounts or ratios you may need.

People will often leap to conclusions and say an herb doesn't work. Well, I'm sorry but if you have almost zero zinc, these herbs can't really make up for that fact. But if you have the bases covered then watch out.

When it comes to testosterone supporting herbs there are lots of options. In my personal experience there are two herbs that work better than anything else I've seen or tried out myself.

Pine Pollen, specifically the tincture form. https://supermanherbs.com/pine-pollen/

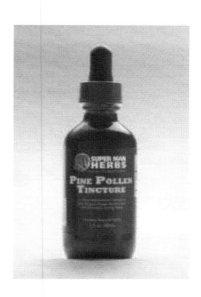
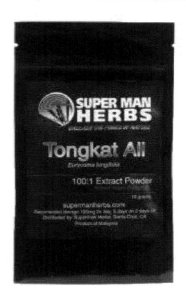

And a potent water extracted Tongkat Ali. https://supermanherbs.com/tongkat-ali/

These work through different mechanisms, but they both to seem to work quite well. If you find yourself at the bottom of a deep hole try taking both at once. Then go out and lift something heavy and you'll be well on your way.

(Personally, because I've gotten more testosterone to levels I'm happy with, I only use these sparingly, because the truth is they're often too powerful for me. I haven't done both at the same time in a long time. But that's because I'm riding a virtuous cycle. For others this may be the best action.)

Of course, it's not just taking these things. There are two more steps that will serve to supercharge these even further. That's because the manner in which we take them also matters.

One of the most fascinating studies about testosterone, and one which helped me to understand the implication that hormones work both ways as chemical messengers was as follows.

This study, *Power Posing: Brief Nonverbal Displays Affect Neuroendocrine Levels and Risk Tolerance*, by Cuddy, Carney and Yap, looked at body language and found that by taking more "dominant" poses testosterone immediately increased, while cortisol went down. And the opposite occurred in "non-dominant" poses.

So what I want you to do while you're taking these nutrients and herbs especially is to do so in a powerful position. Stand or sit like a real man. Erect spine. Head held high. Breathing deeply. Chest held high and shoulders back. See the next page for more examples, as well as what not to do.

This physiology does affect your hormones levels. Of course, you should do it throughout the day, but here we are using it to stack the benefits.

And that's not all. In addition, it is my belief that HOW you think will also affect your hormone levels. If body language affects testosterone, why wouldn't your thoughts? After all, you can think about biting into a lemon and your mouth will begin to pucker and saliva flows. Our body and mind are intimately connected.

While you do this (and really any other practice designed to help your hormones) you want to engage in thoughts about how what you are doing is going to help restore your hormone levels and maximize your manliness.

This can come in different forms. Some people might "feel" the testosterone flowing. Other people may visualize how they're going to act and feel in the future. Still others may imagine seeing numbers having gone up from testing hormones and others asking what they did to do so. Experiment and find what works for you.

The placebo effect is when something that otherwise shouldn't work, does work, because we come to believe in it. Now these nutrients and herbs certainly do work. There is science and plenty of anecdotal evidence behind them. (Not much science behind the pine pollen yet but hopefully there will be soon.) Even so, that doesn't mean we can't supercharge the results by believing in what we're doing on top of it.

In every study averages are what is looked at to achieve statistical significance. But if you look at individuals you can see ones with no or negative results, and those that had phenomenal results. Why not become the high point outlier yourself? Basically you can get a real effect and a so-called placebo effect at the same time.

It's an affirmation or belief that what you're doing is optimizing your hormones. Feed this into your subconscious and the body will better act on it.

It is in stacking these things together you can expect even greater results. Some people will likely note results right away. Others may take some time to do so. Just to recap, do the following:

1. Take Nutrience to make sure all your micronutrient bases are covered.

2. Take Pine Pollen Tincture for a hormonal boost.

3. Take Tongkat Ali for another, albeit different, hormonal boost.

4. Do all these while engage in a high power posture.

5. Do all of these while thinking, visualizing and feeling how what you are doing is going to lead to better hormone levels.

Of course, this can and should be customized to you as an individual. There's many other possible steps you could add in, or substitutions you could make. But armed with this simple five-step formula I feel many men could make dramatic improvements quickly and get into a virtuous cycle.

While the final steps are free the first few take a little money. But for less than $100 a month it's a great deal. With higher testosterone levels it should be easy to make that extra money some way!

Here is the truth about it. These are not just cycles but instead more like a spiral. Whether it goes up or down is largely up to you.

When you're in the virtuous cycle, one of my mentors described it as an "upward expanding spiral of greatness."

Isn't that where you want to be?

Recommended Books

- Carruthers, M., & Carruthers, M. (2001). The testosterone revolution: Rediscover your energy and overcome the symptoms of male menopause. London: Thorsons.
- Buhner, S. H. (2007). The natural testosterone plan: For sexual health and energy. Rochester, VT: Healing Arts Press.
- Hofmekler, O. (2007). *The anti-estrogenic diet: How estrogenic foods and chemicals are making you fat and sick.* Berkeley, CA: North Atlantic Books.
- Miller, P. L., & Reinagel, M. (2005). *The life extension revolution: The new science of growing older without aging.* New York: Bantam Books.
- Shanahan, C., & Shanahan, L. (2009). *Deep nutrition: Why your genes need traditional food.* Lawai, HI: Big Box Books.
- Hill, N. (2016). *Think and grow rich.* Penguin Books.
- Batmanghelidj, F. (1995). *Your body's many cries for water: You are not sick, you are thirsty!: Don't treat thirst with medications.* Falls Church, VA: Global Health Solutions.
- Christopher, L. (2016) *Upgrade Your Breath.* Santa Cruz, CA Legendary Strength Publications
- Christopher, L. (2015) *Upgrade Your Growth Hormone.* Santa Cruz, CA Legendary Strength Publications
- Gottfried, S. (2013). *The hormone cure: Reclaim balance, sleep, sex drive, and vitality naturally with the Gottfried Protocol.* New York, NY: Scribner.
- Bowden, J., & Sinatra, S. T. (2012). *The great cholesterol myth: Why lowering your cholesterol won't prevent heart disease-- and the statin-free plan that will.* Beverly, MA: Fair Winds Press.
- Moore, J., & Westman, E. C. (n.d.). *Cholesterol clarity: What the HDL is wrong with my numbers?*
- Wolfe, D., & Gauthier, R. A. (n.d.). *Longevity now: A comprehensive approach to healthy hormones, detoxification, super immunity, reversing calcification, and total rejuvenation.*
- Winston, S. (2010). *Women's anatomy of arousal: Secret maps to buried pleasure.* Kingston, NY: Mango Garden.

eBooks
- Christopher, L. *Upgrade Your Water* (2014) ebook
- Christopher, L. *Upgrade Your Fat* (2014) ebook
- Christopher, L. *Upgrade Your Sleep* (2014) ebook
- Kuoppala A, *The Secret that Doubles Testosterone* (accessed 2014) ebook
- Walker, C. *Testshock Program: 100% Natural Testosterone Enhancement* (2014) ebook

Scientific References

The Importance of Testosterone

1. Travison, T. G., Araujo, A. B., O'Donnell, A. B., Kupelian, V., & Mckinlay, J. B. (2007). A Population-Level Decline in Serum Testosterone Levels in American Men. The Journal of Clinical Endocrinology & Metabolism, 92(1), 196-202.

How Testosterone, and about 20 Other Hormones, are Created and Converted
2. Häggström, Mikael (2014). "Diagram of the pathways of human steroidogenesis". Wikiversity Journal of Medicine 1 (1). doi:10.15347/wjm/2014.005

The Testosterone Metaphor
3. Vignozzi L, et al. (2005) Testosterone and sexual activity. Journal of endocrinological investigation 28(3 Suppl):39-44.
4. Escasa MJ, Casey JF, & Gray PB (2011) Salivary testosterone levels in men at a U.S. sex club. Archives of sexual behavior 40(5):921-926.
5. Stoléru SG, et al LH pulsatile secretion and testosterone blood levels are influenced by sexual arousal in human males . Psychoneuroendocrinology. (1993)
6. Carney, D. R., Cuddy, A. J., & Yap, A. J. (2010). Power Posing: Brief Nonverbal Displays Affect Neuroendocrine Levels and Risk Tolerance. Psychological Science, 21(10), 1363-1368.
7. Mazur, A., & Booth, A. (1998). Testosterone and dominance in men. Behavioral and Brain Sciences Behav. Brain Sci., 21(03).

Free Testing for Hormone Health
8. Basar, M. M., Atan, A., & Tekdogan, U. Y. (2001). New concept parameters of RigiScan in differentiation of vascular erectile dysfunction: Is it a useful test? International Journal of Urology Int J Urol, 8(12), 686-691.
9. Bancroft, J. (2005). The endocrinology of sexual arousal. Journal of Endocrinology, 186(3), 411-427.
10. Dingfelder, S. (n.d.). Men who cheat show elevated testosterone levels. PsycEXTRA Dataset.

11. O'Carroll R, Shapiro C, & Bancroft J (1985) Androgens, behaviour and nocturnal erection in hypogonadal men: the effects of varying the replacement dose. Clinical endocrinology 23(5):527-538.
12. Montorsi F & Oettel M (2005) Testosterone and sleep-related erections: an overview*. The journal of sexual medicine 2(6):771-784.

Covering the Basics
13. Yildirim, I. (2015). Associations Among Dehydration, Testosterone and Stress Hormones in Terms of Body Weight Loss Before Competition. The American Journal of the Medical Sciences, 350(2), 103-108. Retrieved from
14. Axelsson J, Ingre M, Akerstedt T, & Holmback U (2005) Effects of acutely displaced sleep on testosterone. The Journal of clinical endocrinology and metabolism 90(8):4530-4535.
15. Schiavi RC, White D, & Mandeli J (1992) Pituitary-gonadal function during sleep in healthy aging men. Psychoneuroendocrinology 17(6):599-609.

The Macro-Nutrient Wars
16. Lambert, E. V., & Speechly, D. P. et al. (1994). Enhanced endurance in trained cyclists during moderate intensity exercise following 2 weeks adaptation to a high fat diet. Eur J Appl Physiol European Journal of Applied Physiology and Occupational Physiology, 69(4), 287-293.
17. Anderson, K. E., Rosner, W., Khan, M., New, M. I., Pang, S., Wissel, P. S., & Kappas, A. (1987). Diet-hormone interactions: Protein/carbohydrate ratio alters reciprocally the plasma levels of testosterone and cortisol and their respective binding globulins in man. Life Sciences, 40(18), 1761-1768.
18. Lane, A. R., Duke, J. W., & Hackney, A. C. (2009). Influence of dietary carbohydrate intake on the free testosterone: Cortisol ratio responses to short-term intensive exercise training. European Journal of Applied Physiology Eur J Appl Physiol, 108(6), 1125-1131.

19. Fukushima, M., Watanabe, S., & Kushima, K. (1976). Extraction and Purification of a Substance with Luteinizing Hormone Releasing Activity from the Leaves of Avena sativa. *Tohoku J. Exp. Med. The Tohoku Journal of Experimental Medicine, 119*(2), 115-122.
20. Male pseudohermaphroditism due to steroid 5α-reductase deficiency. (1977). *The American Journal of Medicine, 62*(2).
21. Volek JS, Kraemer WJ, Bush JA, Incledon T, & Boetes M (1997) Testosterone and cortisol in relationship to dietary nutrients and resistance exercise. *Journal of applied physiology* 82(1):49-54.
22. Castellano, C., & Audet, I. (2011). Fish oil diets alter the phospholipid balance, fatty acid composition, and steroid hormone concentrations in testes of adult pigs. *Theriogenology, 76*(6), 1134-1145.
23. Derouiche A, Jafri A, Driouch I, et al. (2013) Effect of argan and olive oil consumption on the hormonal profile of androgens among healthy adult Moroccan men. Nat Prod Commun. 2013 Jan;8(1):51-3.
24. Catalfo, G. E., Alaniz, M. J., & Marra, C. A. (2009). Influence of Commercial Dietary Oils on Lipid Composition and Testosterone Production in Interstitial Cells Isolated from Rat Testis. *Lipids, 44*(4), 345-357.
25. Hamalainen E, Adlercreutz H, Puska P, & Pietinen P (1984) Diet and serum sex hormones in healthy men. *Journal of steroid biochemistry* 20(1):459-464.
26. Ho, K. Y., Veldhuis, J. D., & Johnson, M. L. (1988). Fasting enhances growth hormone secretion and amplifies the complex rhythms of growth hormone secretion in man. *Journal of Clinical Investigation J. Clin. Invest., 81*(4), 968-975.

Limit Endocrine Disruptors
27. Dodds, E. C., Goldberg, L., Lawson, W., & Robinson, R. (1938). Œstrogenic Activity of Certain Synthetic Compounds. *Nature, 141*(3562), 247-248.
28. Sultan, C., Terouanne, B., & Georget, V. et al. (2001). Environmental xenoestrogens, antiandrogens and disorders of male sexual differentiation. *Molecular and Cellular Endocrinology, 178*(1-2), 99-105.
29. Paterni, I., Granchi, C., & Minutolo, F. (2016). Risks and Benefits Related to Alimentary Exposure to Xenoestrogens. *Critical Reviews in Food Science and Nutrition,* 00-00.
30. Mattison, D. R., Karyakina, N., Goodman, M., & Lakind, J. S. (2014). Pharmaco- and toxicokinetics of selected exogenous and endogenous estrogens: A review of the data and identification of knowledge gaps. *Critical Reviews in Toxicology, 44*(8), 696-724.
31. Milligan, S. R. (2000). The Endocrine Activities of 8-Prenylnaringenin and Related Hop (Humulus lupulus L.) Flavonoids. *Journal of Clinical Endocrinology & Metabolism, 85*(12), 4912-4915.
32. Costa, N. O., Vieira, M. L., & Sgarioni, V. et al. (2015). Evaluation of the reproductive toxicity of fungicide propiconazole in male rats. *Toxicology, 335,* 55-61.
33. Guyot, E., Solovyova, Y., & Tomkiewicz, C. (2015). Determination of Heavy Metal Concentrations in Normal and Pathological Human Endometrial Biopsies and In Vitro Regulation of Gene Expression by Metals in the Ishikawa and Hec-1b Endometrial Cell Line. *PLOS ONE PLoS ONE, 10*(11).
34. Videmann, B., & Mazallon, M. et al. (2009). ABCC1, ABCC2 and ABCC3 are implicated in the transepithelial transport of the myco-estrogen zearalenone and its major metabolites. *Toxicology Letters, 190*(2), 215-223.
35. Ruyck, K. D., Boevre, M. D., Huybrechts, I., & Saeger, S. D. (2015). Dietary mycotoxins, co-exposure, and carcinogenesis in humans: Short review. *Mutation Research/Reviews in Mutation Research, 766,* 32-41.
36. Luzio, A., Monteiro, S. M., & Rocha, E et al. (2016). Development and recovery of histopathological alterations in the gonads of zebrafish (Danio rerio) after single and combined exposure to endocrine disruptors (17α-ethinylestradiol and fadrozole). *Aquatic Toxicology, 175,* 90-105.

Detox Endocrine Disruptors
37. Comhaire, F. H., & Depypere, H. T. (2015). Hormones, herbal preparations and nutriceuticals for a better life after the menopause: Part I. *Climacteric, 18*(3), 358-363.
38. Gonzales, G. (2003). Effect of Lepidium meyenii (Maca), a root with aphrodisiac and fertility-enhancing properties, on serum reproductive hormone levels in adult healthy men. *Journal of Endocrinology, 176*(1), 163-168.

39. Michnovicz, J. J., Adlercreutz, H., & Bradlow, H. L. (1997). Changes in Levels of Urinary Estrogen Metabolites After Oral Indole-3-Carbinol Treatment in Humans. *JNCI Journal of the National Cancer Institute, 89*(10), 718-723.

40. Wang, T. T., Schoene, N. W., Milner, J. A., & Kim, Y. S. (2011). Broccoli-derived phytochemicals indole-3-carbinol and 3,3'-diindolylmethane exerts concentration-dependent pleiotropic effects on prostate cancer cells: Comparison with other cancer preventive phytochemicals. Mol. Carcinog. Molecular Carcinogenesis, 51(3), 244-256.

41. Ravoori, S., Vadhanam, M. V., Aqil, F., & Gupta, R. C. (2012). Inhibition of Estrogen-Mediated Mammary Tumorigenesis by Blueberry and Black Raspberry. *J. Agric. Food Chem. Journal of Agricultural and Food Chemistry, 60*(22), 5547-5555.

42. Walaszek, Z. (1990). Potential use of d-glucaric acid derivatives in cancer prevention. *Cancer Letters, 54*(1-2), 1-8.

43. Rajdl, D., Trefil, L., & Babuska, V. (2016). Effect of Folic Acid, Betaine, Vitamin B6, and Vitamin B12 on Homocysteine and Dimethylglycine Levels in Middle-Aged Men Drinking White Wine. *Nutrients, 8*(1), 34.

44. Ejaz, A., Martinez-Guino, L., & Goldfine, A. B. et al. (2016). Dietary Betaine Supplementation Increases Fgf21 Levels to Improve Glucose Homeostasis and Reduce Hepatic Lipid Accumulation in Mice. *Diabetes, 65*(4), 902-912.

45. Jahan, S., Ain, Q. U., & Ullah, H. (2016). Therapeutic effects of quercetin against bisphenol A induced testicular damage in male Sprague Dawley rats. *Systems Biology in Reproductive Medicine, 62*(2), 114-124.

46. Truan, J. S., Chen, J., & Thompson, L. U. (2012). Comparative Effects of Sesame Seed Lignan and Flaxseed Lignan in Reducing the Growth of Human Breast Tumors (MCF-7) at High Levels of Circulating Estrogen in Athymic Mice. *Nutrition and Cancer, 64*(1), 65-71.

Lower Cortisol

47. Ponzi, D., Zilioli, S., & Mehta, P. H. (2016). Social network centrality and hormones: The interaction of testosterone and cortisol. *Psychoneuroendocrinology, 68*, 6-13.

48. Sherman, G. D., Lerner, J. S., & Josephs, R. A. (2015). The Interaction of Testosterone and Cortisol Is Associated With Attained Status in Male Executives. *Journal of Personality and Social Psychology*.

49. Yoo, Y., Lee, D., & Lee, I. et al. (2016). The Effects of Mind Subtraction Meditation on Depression, Social Anxiety, Aggression, and Salivary Cortisol Levels of Elementary School Children in South Korea. *Journal of Pediatric Nursing*.

50. Lau, W. K., Leung, M., & Chan, C. C. et al. (2015). Can the neural–cortisol association be moderated by experience-induced changes in awareness? *Sci. Rep. Scientific Reports, 5*, 16620.

51. Robert-Mccomb, J. J., Cisneros, A., & Tacón, A. (2015). The Effects of Mindfulness-Based Movement on Parameters of Stress. *International Journal of Yoga Therapy, 25*(1), 79-88.

52. White, C. S. (n.d.). The Impact Of Self-Practice Qigong On Strength Gains And Wellbeing During Off-Season Training For Fall Sport Athletes.

53. Panossian, A., Wikman, G., Kaur, P., & Asea, A. (2009). Adaptogens exert a stress-protective effect by modulation of expression of molecular chaperones. *Phytomedicine, 16*(6-7), 617-622.

54. Enwonwu, C., Sawiris, P., & Chanaud, N. (1995). Effect of marginal ascorbic acid deficiency on saliva level of cortisol in the guinea pig. *Archives of Oral Biology, 40*(8), 737-742.

Lower Aromatase

55. Polari, L., Yatkin, E., & Chacón, M. (2015). Weight gain and inflammation regulate aromatase expression in male adipose tissue, as evidenced by reporter gene activity. *Molecular and Cellular Endocrinology, 412*, 123-130.

56. Li, W., Pandey, A. K., Yin, X., & Chen, J. (2011). Effects of apigenin on steroidogenesis and steroidogenic acute regulatory gene expression in mouse Leydig cells. *The Journal of Nutritional Biochemistry, 22*(3), 212-218.

57. Lu, D., Yang, L., Wang, F., & Zhang, G. (2012). Inhibitory Effect of Luteolin on Estrogen Biosynthesis in Human Ovarian Granulosa Cells by Suppression of Aromatase (CYP19). *J. Agric. Food Chem. Journal of Agricultural and Food Chemistry, 60*(34), 8411-8418.

58. Chen, S., Oh, S., Phung, S., & Hur, G. (2006). Anti-Aromatase Activity of Phytochemicals in White Button Mushrooms (Agaricus bisporus). *Cancer Research, 66*(24), 12026-12034.

59. Kao, Y. C., Zhou, C., Sherman, M., Laughton, C. A., & Chen, S. (1998). Molecular basis of the inhibition of human aromatase (estrogen synthetase) by flavone and isoflavone phytoestrogens: A site-directed mutagenesis study. *Environ Health Perspect Environmental Health Perspectives, 106*(2), 85-92.

60. Subbaramaiah, K., Sue, E., & Bhardwaj, P. (2013). Dietary Polyphenols Suppress Elevated Levels of Proinflammatory Mediators and Aromatase in the Mammary Gland of Obese Mice. *Cancer Prevention Research, 6*(9), 886-897.

61. Neves, M. A., Dinis, T. C., Colombo, G., & Melo, M. L. (2007). Combining Computational and Biochemical Studies for a Rationale on the Anti-Aromatase Activity of Natural Polyphenols. *ChemMedChem, 2*(12), 1750-1762.

62. Chrubasik, J. E., Roufogalis, B. D., Wagner, H., & Chrubasik, S. (2007). A comprehensive review on the stinging nettle effect and efficacy profiles. Part II: Urticae radix. *Phytomedicine, 14*(7-8), 568-579.

63. Low, B., Choi, S., & Wahab, H. A. (2013). Eurycomanone, the major quassinoid in Eurycoma longifolia root extract increases spermatogenesis by inhibiting the activity of phosphodiesterase and aromatase in steroidogenesis. *Journal of Ethnopharmacology, 149*(1), 201-207.

Lower SHBG

64. Reed, M., Cheng, R., Simmonds, M., Richmond, W., & James, V. (1987). Dietary Lipids: An Additional Regulator Of Plasma Levels Of Sex Hormone Binding Globulin. The Journal of Clinical Endocrinology & Metabolism, 64(5), 1083-1085.

65. Kappas, A., Anderson, K. E., & Conney, A. H. (1983). Nutrition-endocrine interactions: Induction of reciprocal changes in the delta 4-5 alpha-reduction of testosterone and the cytochrome P-450-dependent oxidation of estradiol by dietary macronutrients in man. *Proceedings of the National Academy of Sciences, 80*(24), 7646-7649.

66. Iturriaga, H. (1999). Sex Hormone-Binding Globulin In Non-Cirrhotic Alcoholic Patients During Early Withdrawal And After Longer Abstinence. Alcohol and Alcoholism, 34(6), 903-909.

67. Nagata, C., Takatsuka, N., Kawakami, N., & Shimizu, H. (2000). Relationships Between Types of Fat Consumed and SerumEstrogen and Androgen Concentrations in Japanese Men. *Nutrition and Cancer, 38*(2), 163-167.

68. Excoffon, L., Guillaume, Y., Woronoff-Lemsi, M., & André, C. (2009). Magnesium effect on testosterone–SHBG association studied by a novel molecular chromatography approach. *Journal of Pharmaceutical and Biomedical Analysis, 49*(2), 175-180.

69. Schöttner, M., Ganßer, D., & Spiteller, G. (1997). Lignans from the Roots of Urtica dioica and their Metabolites Bind to Human Sex Hormone Binding Globulin (SHBG). Planta Med Planta Medica, 63(06), 529-532.

Lower Prolactin

70. Shukla, K. K., Mahdi, A. A., Ahmad, M. K., Shankhwar, S. N., Rajender, S., & Jaiswar, S. P. (2009). Mucuna pruriens improves male fertility by its action on the hypothalamus–pituitary–gonadal axis. Fertility and Sterility, 92(6), 1934-1940.

71. Delvecchio, M., Faienza, M. F., Lonero, A., & Rutigliano, V. (2014). Prolactin May Be Increased in Newly Diagnosed Celiac Children and Adolescents and Decreases after 6 Months of Gluten-Free Diet. *Horm Res Paediatr Hormone Research in Paediatrics, 81*(5), 309-313.

72. Mahdi, A. A., Shukla, K. K., & Ahmad, M. K. (2011). Withania somnifera Improves Semen Quality in Stress-Related Male Fertility. *Evidence-Based Complementary and Alternative Medicine, 2011*, 1-9.

73. Delitala, G., Masala, A., Alagna, S., & Devilla, L. (1976). Effect Of Pyridoxine On Human Hypophyseal Trophic Hormone Release: A Possible Stimulation Of Hypothalamic Dopaminergic Pathway. *The Journal of Clinical Endocrinology & Metabolism, 42*(3), 603-606.

74. Néto, J., Mendonça, B. D., & Shuhama, T. (1989). Zinc: An Inhibitor of Prolactin (PRL) Secretion in Humans. *Hormone and Metabolic Research Horm Metab Res, 21*(04), 203-206.

Cholesterol

75. Keyser, C. E., Lima, F. V., & Jong, F. H. et al. (2015). Use of statins is associated with lower serum total and non-sex hormone-binding globulin-bound testosterone levels in male participants of the Rotterdam Study. *Eur J Endocrinol European Journal of Endocrinology, 173*(2), 155-165.

76. Freedman, D. S., O'brien, T. R., Flanders, W. D., Destefano, F., & Barboriak, J. J. (1991). Relation of serum testosterone levels to high density lipoprotein cholesterol and other characteristics in men. *Arteriosclerosis, Thrombosis, and Vascular Biology, 11*(2), 307-315.

77. Wang, C., Catlin, D. H., & Starcevic, B. (2005). Low-Fat High-Fiber Diet Decreased Serum and Urine Androgens in Men. *The Journal of Clinical Endocrinology & Metabolism, 90*(6), 3550-3559.

Micronutrients

78. Prasad, A. (1996). Zinc Status and Serum Testosterone Levels of Healthy Adults. Nutrition, 12(5), Vi.

79. Netter, A., Nahoul, K., & Hartoma, R. (1981). Effect of Zinc Administration on Plasma Testosterone, Dihydrotestosterone, and Sperm Count. *Archives of Andrology, 7*(1), 69-73.

80. Jalali, G., Roozbeh, J., & Mohammadzadeh, A. (2010). Impact of oral zinc therapy on the level of sex hormones in male patients on hemodialysis. *Renal Failure, 32*(4), 417-419.

81. Domingo, V., Prieto, C., & Silva, L. (2016). Iodine, a Mild Reagent for the Aromatization of Terpenoids. *J. Nat. Prod. Journal of Natural Products*.

82. Cai, J., Wang, C., & Wu, T. (2011). Disruption of spermatogenesis and differential regulation of testicular estrogen receptor expression in mice after polychlorinated biphenyl exposure. *Toxicology, 287*(1-3), 21-28.

83. Chakraborty, A., Mandal, J., & Mondal, C. (2015). Effect of Excess Iodine on Oxidative Stress Markers, Steroidogenic—Enzyme Activities, Testicular Morphology, and Functions in Adult Male Rats. *Biological Trace Element Research Biol Trace Elem Res*.

84. Naghii, M. R., Mofid, M., & Asgari, A. R. et al. (2011). Comparative effects of daily and weekly boron supplementation on plasma steroid hormones and proinflammatory cytokines. *Journal of Trace Elements in Medicine and Biology, 25*(1), 54-58.

85. Dupre, J. N., Keenan, M. J., Hegsted, M., & Brudevold, A. M. (1994). Effects of Dietary Boron in Rats Fed a Vitamin D-Deficient Diet. *Environmental Health Perspectives, 102*, 55.

86. Bishop, D. T., Meikle, A. W., & Slattery, M. L. (1988). The effect of nutritional factors on sex hormone levels in male twins. *Genetic Epidemiology Genet. Epidemiol., 5*(1), 43-59.

87. Umeda, F., Kato, K., Muta, K., & Ibayashi, H. (1982). Effect of vitamin E on function of pituitary-gonadal axis in male rats and human subjects. *Endocrinologia Japonica Endocrinol Japon, 29*(3), 287-292.

88. Ito, A., Shirakawa, H., & Takumi, N. (2011). Menaquinone-4 enhances testosterone production in rats and testis-derived tumor cells. *Lipids Health Dis Lipids in Health and Disease, 10*(1), 158.

89. Cinar, V., Polat, Y., Baltaci, A. K., & Mogulkoc, R. (2010). Effects of Magnesium Supplementation on Testosterone Levels of Athletes and Sedentary Subjects at Rest and after Exhaustion. *Biological Trace Element Research Biol Trace Elem Res, 140*(1), 18-23.

Sunshine and Vitamin D

90. Holick MF (2016). Biological Effects of Sunlight, Ultraviolet Radiation, Visible Light, Infrared Radiation and Vitamin D for Health. Anticancer Res. 36(3):1345-56.

91. Wehr, E., Pilz, S., Boehm, B., Mä□Rz, W., & Obermayer-Pietsch, B. (2009). Association of vitamin D status with serum androgen levels in men. Clinical Endocrinology.

92. Pilz, S., Frisch, S., Koertke, H., Kuhn, J., Dreier, J., Obermayer-Pietsch, B., Zittermann, A. (2010). Effect of Vitamin D Supplementation on Testosterone Levels in Men. Hormone and Metabolic Research Horm Metab Res, 43(03), 223-225.

Cell Receptor Health

93. Ceccarelli, C., Canale, D., & Vitti, P. (2008). Radioactive iodine (131I) effects on male fertility. *Current Opinion in Urology, 18*(6), 598-601.

Increase LH and Other T Precursors

94. Waleed Abid Al-Kadir Mares, Wisam S. Najam (2012). The effect of Ginger on semen parameters and serum FSH, LH &testosterone of infertile men, 18(2), 322-329.

95. Bakrim, A., Maria, A., & Sayah, F. (2008). Ecdysteroids in spinach (Spinacia oleracea L.): Biosynthesis, transport and regulation of levels. *Plant Physiology and Biochemistry, 46*(10), 844-854.

96. Sidorova I., Seliaskin K., Zorin S., (2014) Phytoecdysteroids influence on the hormonal status and apoptosis in growing rats Vopr Pitan. 83(2):16-21.

97. Gorelick-Feldman, J., Maclean, D., & Ilic, N. (2008). Phytoecdysteroids Increase Protein Synthesis in Skeletal Muscle Cells. *J. Agric. Food Chem. Journal of Agricultural and Food Chemistry, 56*(10), 3532-3537.

98. Graf, B. L., Rojo, L. E., & Delatorre-Herrera, J. (2015). Phytoecdysteroids and flavonoid glycosides among Chilean and commercial sources of Chenopodium quinoa : Variation and correlation to physico-chemical characteristics. *Journal of the Science of Food and Agriculture J. Sci. Food Agric., 96*(2), 633-643.

99. George, A., & Henkel, R. (2014). Phytoandrogenic properties of Eurycoma longifolia as natural alternative to testosterone replacement therapy. *Andrologia, 46*(7), 708-721.

Increase Testosterone Directly

100. Šaden-Krehula, M., Tajić, M., & Kolbah, D. (1971). Testosterone, epitestosterone and androstenedione in the pollen of scotch pineP. silvestris L. *Experientia, 27*(1), 108-109.

101. Bernhardt, P. C., Jr, J. M., Fielden, J. A., & Lutter, C. D. (1998). Testosterone changes during vicarious experiences of winning and losing among fans at sporting events. Physiology & Behavior, 65(1), 59-62.

102. Seo, Y., Jeong, B., Kim, J., & Choi, J. (2009). Plasma Concentration of Prolactin, Testosterone Might Be Associated with Brain Response to Visual Erotic Stimuli in Healthy Heterosexual Males. *Psychiatry Investigation Psychiatry Investig, 6*(3), 194.

DHT

103. Chiriacò, G., Cauci, S., Mazzon, G., & Trombetta, C. (2016). An observational retrospective evaluation of 79 young men with long-term adverse effects after use of finasteride against androgenetic alopecia. *Andrology, 4*(2), 245-250.

104. Catalona, W. (1995). Evaluation of percentage of free serum prostate-specific antigen to improve specificity of prostate cancer screening. *JAMA: The Journal of the American Medical Association,* 1214-1220.

105. Carter, H., Pearson, J., Metter, E., Chan, D., Andres, R., Fozard, J., . . . Walsh, P. (n.d.). Longitudinal evaluation of serum androgen levels in men with and without prostate cancer. *The Prostate Prostate,* 25-31.

106. Morgentaler, A. (1996). Occult prostate cancer in men with low serum testosterone levels. *JAMA: The Journal of the American Medical Association,*1904-1906.

107. Ghanadian, R., & Puah, C. (n.d.). The clinical significance of steroid hormone measurements in the management of patients with prostatic cancer. *World J Urol World Journal of Urology,* 49-54.

108. Suzuki, K., Ito, K., Ichinose, Y., Kurokawa, K., Suzuki, T., Imai, K., . . . Honma, S. (n.d.). Endocrine Environment of Benign Prostatic Hyperplasia: Prostate Size and Volume are Correlated with Serum Estrogen Concentration. *Scand J Urol Nephrol Scandinavian Journal of Urology and Nephrology,* 65-68.

109. Bosland, M., & Mahmoud, A. (n.d.). Hormones and prostate carcinogenesis: Androgens and estrogens. *Journal of Carcinogenesis J Carcinog,* 33-33.

110. Cheng, H., & Montgomery, B. (n.d.). Androgen Receptor Biology in Castration Resistant Prostate Cancer. *Management of Castration Resistant Prostate Cancer Current Clinical Urology,* 67-75.

111. Moreel, X., Allaire, J., Leger, C., Caron, A., Labonte, M., Lamarche, B., . . . Fradet, V. (2014). Prostatic and Dietary Omega-3 Fatty Acids and Prostate Cancer Progression during Active Surveillance. *Cancer Prevention Research,*766-776.

112. Manuel J., Schottker B., Fedirko V. et al. (2015) Pre-diagnostic vitamin D concentrations and cancer risks in older individuals: an analysis of cohorts participating in the CHANCES consortium. *European Journal of Epidemiology*

113. Leslie C Costello Renty B Franklin. (n.d.). Evidence that Human Prostate Cancer is a ZIP1-Deficient Malignancy that could be Effectively Treated with a Zinc Ionophore (Clioquinol) Approach. *Chemotherapy (Los Angel) Chemotherapy: Open Access*.

114. Macdonald, R., Tacklind, J., Rutks, I., & Wilt, T. (2012). Serenoa repens monotherapy for benign prostatic hyperplasia (BPH): An updated Cochrane systematic review. *BJU International*, 1756-1761.

115. Safarinejad, M. (n.d.). Urtica dioica for Treatment of Benign Prostatic Hyperplasia. *Journal of Herbal Pharmacotherapy*, 1-11.

116. Sökeland, J. (n.d.). Combined sabal and urtica extract compared with finasteride in men with benign prostatic hyperplasia: Analysis of prostate volume and therapeutic outcome. *BJU International*, 439-442.

117. Poole, C., Bushey, B., & Foster, C. (2010). The effects of a commercially available botanical supplement on strength, body composition, power output, and hormonal profiles in resistance-trained males. *J Int Soc Sports Nutr Journal of the International Society of Sports Nutrition, 7*(1), 34.

118. Wang, T., Chen, C., & Yang, M. (2015). Cistanche tubulosa ethanol extract mediates rat sex hormone levels by induction of testicular steroidgenic enzymes. *Pharmaceutical Biology, 54*(3), 481-487.

Establish a Healthy Relationship with Your Cock and Balls

119. Al-Asmakh, M., Stukenborg, J., & Reda, A. (2014). The Gut Microbiota and Developmental Programming of the Testis in Mice. *PLoS ONE, 9*(8).

120. Markle, J. G., Frank, D. N., & Mortin-Toth, S. (2013). Sex Differences in the Gut Microbiome Drive Hormone-Dependent Regulation of Autoimmunity. *Science, 339*(6123), 1084-1088.

121. Sapra, K. J., Eisenberg, M. L., & Kim, S. (2016). Choice of underwear and male fecundity in a preconception cohort of couples. *Andrology*.

122. Lue, Y. (2000). Testicular Heat Exposure Enhances the Suppression of Spermatogenesis by Testosterone in Rats: The "Two-Hit" Approach to Male Contraceptive Development. Endocrinology, 141(4), 1414-1424.

123. Jung, A., & Schuppe, H. (2007). Influence of genital heat stress on semen quality in humans. *Andrologia, 39*(6), 203-215.

124. Myerson, A., & Neustadt, R. (1939). Influence Of Ultraviolet Irradiation Upon Excretion Of Sex Hormones In The Male1 1. *Endocrinology, 25*(1), 7-12.

125. Zhang, G., Yan, H., & Chen, Q. (2016). Effects of cell phone use on semen parameters: Results from the MARHCS cohort study in Chongqing, China. *Environment International, 91*, 116-121.

T-Boosting Workouts

[1] Shrier, I. (2007). Differential effects of strength training leading to failure versus not to failure on hormonal responses, strength, and muscle power gains. Yearbook of Sports Medicine, 2007, 99-100.

[2] Gotshalk, L. A., Loebel, C. C., & Nindl, B. C. et al. (1997). Hormonal Responses of Multiset Versus Single-Set Heavy-Resistance Exercise Protocols. *Canadian Journal of Applied Physiology Can. J. Appl. Physiol., 22*(3), 244-255.

[3] Rahimi, R., Ghaderi, M., & Mirzaei, B. et al. (2010). Effects of very short rest periods on immunoglobulin A and cortisol responses to resistance exercise in men. *Journal of Human Sport and Exercise Jhse, 5*(2), 146-157.

[4] Rosa, C., Vilaça-Alves, J., & Fernandes, H. M. et al. (2015). Order Effects of Combined Strength and Endurance Training on Testosterone, Cortisol, Growth Hormone, and IGF-1 Binding Protein 3 in Concurrently Trained Men. *Journal of Strength and Conditioning Research, 29*(1), 74-79.

[5] Ahtiainen, J. P., Pakarinen, A., Kraemer, W. J., & Hakkinen, K. (2004). Acute Hormonal Responses to Heavy Resistance Exercise in Strength Athletes Versus Nonathletes. *Canadian Journal of Applied Physiology Can. J. Appl. Physiol., 29*(5), 527-543.

[6] Shaner, A. A., Vingren, J. L., & Hatfield, D. L. (2014). The Acute Hormonal Response to Free Weight and Machine Weight Resistance Exercise. *Journal of Strength and Conditioning Research, 28*(4), 1032-1040.

[7] Trumble, B. C., O'Connor, K. A., & Smith, E. A. et al. (2013). Age-independent increases in male salivary testosterone during horticultural activity among Tsimane forager-farmers. *Evolution and Human Behavior, 34*(5), 350-357.

[8] West, D. W., & Phillips, S. M. (2010). Anabolic Processes in Human Skeletal Muscle: Restoring the Identities of Growth Hormone and Testosterone. *The Physician and Sportsmedicine, 38*(3), 97-104.

[9] Budnar, R. G., Duplanty, A. A., & Hill, D. W. et al. (2014). The Acute Hormonal Response to the Kettlebell Swing Exercise. *Journal of Strength and Conditioning Research, 28*(10), 2793-2800.

[10] Sato, K., Iemitsu, M., & Matsutani, K. et al. (2014). Resistance training restores muscle sex steroid hormone steroidogenesis in older men. The FASEB Journal, 28(4), 1891-1897.

[11] Cook, C. J., & Beaven, C. M. (2013). Salivary testosterone is related to self-selected training load in elite female athletes. Physiology & Behavior, 116-117, 8-12.

[12] Ghigiarelli, J. J., Sell, K. M., Raddock, J. M., & Taveras, K. (2013). Effects of Strongman Training on Salivary Testosterone Levels in a Sample of Trained Men. Journal of Strength and Conditioning Research, 27(3), 738-747.

[13] Ahtiainen, J. P., Pakarinen, A., Alen, M., et al. (2005). Short vs. Long Rest Period Between the Sets in Hypertrophic Resistance Training: Influence on Muscle Strength, Size, and Hormonal Adaptations in Trained Men. J Strength Cond Res The Journal of Strength and Conditioning Research, 19(3), 572.

About the Author

Born without genetic gifts, a weak and scrawny Logan Christopher sought out the best training information in his pursuit of super strength, mind power and radiant health. Nowadays, he's known for his famous feats of pulling an 8,800 lb. firetruck by his hair, juggling flaming kettlebells, and supporting half a ton in the wrestler's bridge. Called the "Physical Culture Renaissance Man" his typical workouts might include backflips, freestanding handstand pushups, tearing phonebooks in half, bending steel, deadlifting a heavy barbell, or lifting rocks overhead.

Far from being all brawn and no brain Logan has sought optimal performance with mental training and sports psychology which he has explored in depth, becoming an NLP Trainer, certified hypnotist, EFT practitioner and more. That's also how he got started in the field of health and nutrition which inevitably led to Chinese, Ayurvedic and Western herbalism.

His personal philosophy is to bring together the best movement skill, health information, and mental training to achieve peak performance. He is the author of many books and video programs to help people increase their strength, skills, health and mental performance. Discover how you too can become super strong, both mentally and physically, at www.LegendaryStrength.com and find the superior herbs to support all aspects of your performance at www.SuperManHerbs.com.

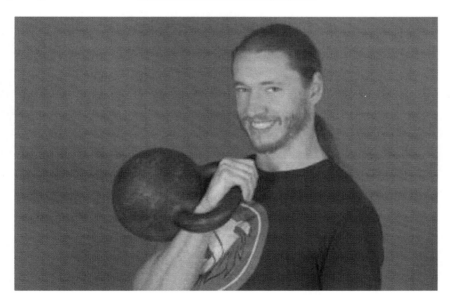

Other Books in the Upgrade Your Health Series:

Upgrade Your Breath http://legendarystrength.com/breath/

Upgrade Your Growth Hormone http://legendarystrength.com/growth-hormone/

Upgrade Your Water http://legendarystrength.com/upgrade-your-water/

Upgrade Your Sleep http://legendarystrength.com/upgrade-your-sleep/

Upgrade Your Fat http://legendarystrength.com/upgrade-your-fat/

Upgrade Your Vitamins http://legendarystrength.com/upgrade-your-vitamins/

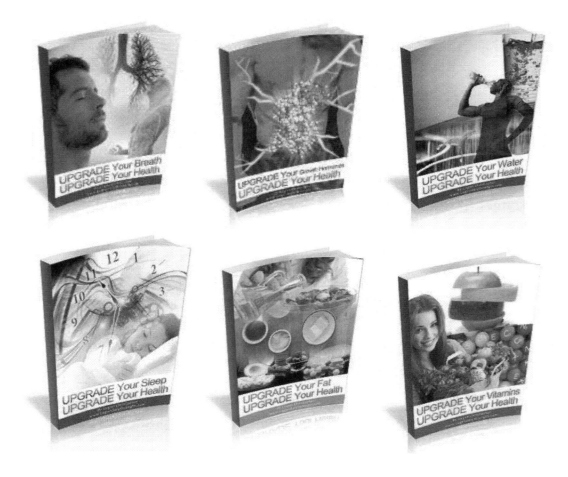

For a full up-to-date of titles in the Upgrade Your Health Series plus more books and videos from Logan Christopher go to:
http://www.LegendaryStrength.com/books-videos/

"Get Stronger... Move Better...
Become Healthier... Unleash Your Mind Power...
Every Single Month"

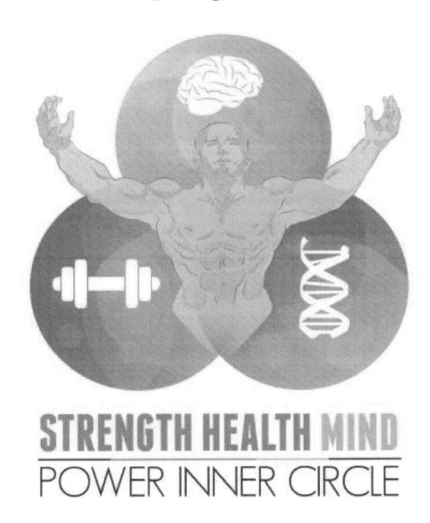

- Monthly Newsletter on Achieving Peak Health & Performance
- Access to Coaching from Logan Christopher
- Private Community of Members
- Free Bonuses and Videos
- And Much More

Go to www.StrengthHealthMindPower.com

Made in the USA
Middletown, DE
04 July 2021

43568526R00091